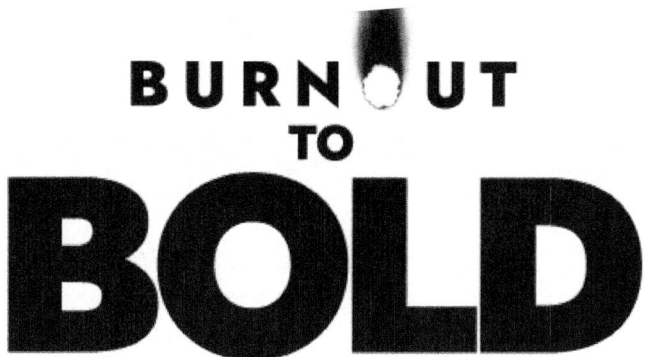

From a flickering light
to a bold flame

Marie Jenkins

Burnout to BOLD

Burnout to Bold: From a flickering light to a bold flame by Marie Jenkins

First Edition (2021)

Copyright © 2012 Marie Jenkins

All rights reserved.

No part of this publication may be reproduced, stored in a retrieval system, or transmitted in any form or by any means without the prior written permission of the publisher and author.

ISBN: 9798545161317

Published by

Albern Publishing

Cover Design: Steve Pitt from Steven Pitt Graphic Design

https://www.stevepitt.com/

Image and Photography by Julie King from Julie King Photography

DEDICATION

This book is for my mom and dad who are no longer with us and had a massive impact on who I am and what has shaped me over my life.

For my three beautiful Children, who have grown into strong resilient adults and who I am proud of every single day.

For my husband Drew, that has shared this journey and helped me realise that I can achieve my true potential.

Finally, my best friend Bourbon, our Springer Spaniel dog, who has listened to all my thoughts and supported me in my dark moments and who I love unconditionally.

Burnout to Bold

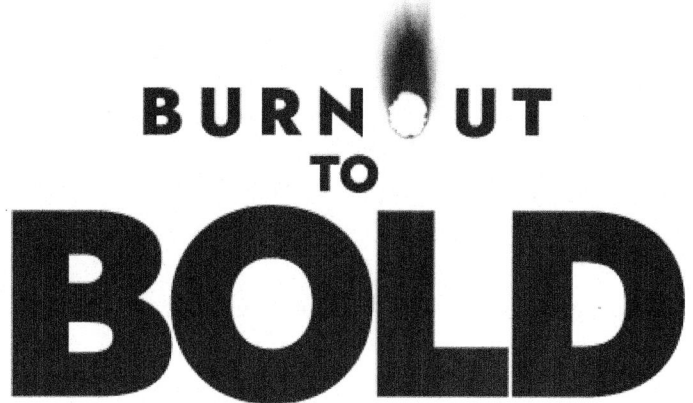

MARIE JENKINS

"A refreshing real-life account, Marie is soft-heartedly honest and open in describing her experience of poor mental health and its devastating effect on her health & wellbeing.

Everyone has experienced poor mental health in their lives to some degree and you will benefit from reading this book. It is crammed with practical advice on how step by step it is possible to build your confidence and self-esteem, prioritise your wellbeing without guilt and to reach out for support and encouragement. It also delves into subjects such as Mindfulness, Emotional Intelligence, and mindset.

The combination of great advice from someone who has been there, together with incredibly useful information as to the resources available makes for invaluable reading.

Discover how Marie transformed her life from feelings of ultimate desperation and worthlessness to a woman who is now a strong bold human being, running her own business, helping others through wellbeing coaching and training in numerous interpersonal skills topics and who just loves to go out cycling at every opportunity!"

Kathy Scott, Hands on at Work and Author of 'Rubbing Shoulders with the Best'.

Burnout to Bold

CONTENTS

CHAPTER 1: MENTAL HEALTH   **13**
- My Story   13
- Today's Environment   23
- Reassessing your Priorities   27
- Things you could explore further   29

My Ditty: The day my Wellies saved me   **35**

CHAPTER 2: 5 WAYS TO WELLBEING   **41**
- Be Active   41
- Keep Learning   44
- Connect   47
- Take notice   49
- Give   52

My Ditty: I cycled a Monkey   **57**

CHAPTER 3: CONFIDENCE & SELF ESTEEM   **65**
- Confidence & Self Esteem   65
- Confidence & Over confidence   66
- Comfort Zone   82
- Reflection   83

My Ditty: Egg on my face   **85**

CHAPTER 4: MINDFULLNESS   **89**
- What is Mindfulness?   89
- How you react and over reaction   90
- Accepting difference and tolerance   91
- Practical ways to use mindfulness techniques   93

My Ditty: The horse has bolted   **109**

CHAPTER 5: RESILIENCE CHILDHOOD   **113**
- Childhood   115
- Values and Beliefs   116
- 5 Pillars of Resilience   117
- Positivity & Facing Your Fears   120

My Ditty: Blood in the Swimming Bath   **125**

CHAPTER 6: EMOTIONAL INTELLIGENCE   **129**

   EQ and Science   129
   Self-Awareness   131
   Self-Management Strategies   133
   Social Awareness   136
   Relationships   139

   My Ditty: The winner is....   **143**

CHAPTER 7: MANAGING CHANGE   **147**

   Mindset   147
   Opportunities or Challenge   149
   Major Life Changes   150
   Innovation   153

   My Ditty: Face of a clown   **157**

CHAPTER 8: LEADERSHIP   **161**

   Leadership Styles   162
   Leadership Voice   164
   Characteristics   165
   Inspiration   166

   My Ditty: Let's do this   **167**

CHAPTER 9: SUPPORT COACHING   **171**

   What is Coaching?   172
   Questioning Techniques   173
   Coaching Models   174
   What is Mentoring?   175
   Mentoring or Coaching   176

   My Ditty: Jumping for Joy   **177**

Appendices   **182**

   Supplementary Resources   182

   Bibliography   184

   Oher Sources   186

   References   188

ACKNOWLEDGEMENTS

Kathy Scott from Hands on at Work for the encouragement to write my first book and for giving me her honest feedback on my first draft.

Vicky Fraser from Moxie Books for giving me all the tools and support needed to get my thoughts into a readable book, that I hope people will want to read.

Steve Pitt, from Steve Pitt Graphic Design for designing a book cover that is eye-catching and stands out on a bookshelf.

Ali Bagley from Ali Bagley Coaching for her dedication to getting my draft into a readable format through to publishing and holding my hand every step of the way.

Thanks to the **SME Community in Worcestershire** and everyone else who has given me the encouragement and belief in my business which has led to my first book.

Julie King from Julie King Photography for the great image used on the back cover, taken in her gorgeous garden.

INTRODUCTION

This book is designed to be part of your mental wellbeing tool kit. Helping you to thrive in today's world, become your better self, and maintain positive mental health.

The topics covered here are key things that I learned about as I recovered from my own mental health battles, and which led me to create my own Wellbeing training business. By sharing my real-life reflections and experiences you will realise that you are not alone, and that you too can achieve your full potential.

You will find a pick and mix of varying topics to improve your interpersonal skills, some that you will find more relevant than others to your personal situation. Whatever your needs are, the content of this book has been designed to move you forward as a more balanced and mentally heathy person.

The beauty of this book is that you can refer to it for support in multiple situations and challenges in your life and career. Wellbeing is something we often take for granted and my desire is that these pages will support you in your continual commitment and dedication to your self-care and mental health throughout your life.

Based on research demonstrating the close correlation between physical health and mental health taking responsibility for your physical health can have positive impacts on your mental wellbeing. This is something that features significantly in the book.

As you read you will find help for your own personal development journey and tools to increase your self-belief, so that you can achieve your full potential in your life and career.

Plus, I share with you some of my own personal Ditty's, stories from my past that have shaped my life and progress. Some will make you laugh, others help you to reflect on your own personal stories, so you know that you, like me, can survive and move forward.

Burnout to Bold

CHAPTER 1: MENTAL HEALTH

At the end of 2013 I was a Head of Service in a local Housing Association, I had a beautiful family and to outsiders I looked like I had the perfect life.

In reality I was struggling with my mental health, was morbidly obese, and I had anxiety and depression to the point where I was on the brink of taking my own life.

I had not been taking responsibility for my own health and wellbeing during a time when I was taking care of my terminally ill mom, at work I was dealing with restructure and redundancies, and at home I was being a mom to three teenage kids.

Everyone else came first before me. Selfcare was a luxury, I could ill afford, or that is what I thought.

I was trying my hardest to juggle all these responsibilities. As a single mom with three beautiful children with ages ranging from 10 - 18yrs I was trying to multitask, so that their lives could run smoothly, being a school liaison, taxi service, cook, and chief bottle washer.

My mom's condition was deteriorating. She had a chronic lung disease, which meant I was coordinating her care following numerous admissions and discharges into and out of hospital. I was liaising between my mom and her support services trying to ensure she was getting the help and support she needed. Just the smallest of tasks would exhaust her, so she needed the maximum help I could give. My phone was constantly ringing.

Burnout to BOLD

The 4 services I was managing as part of my role as a Head of Service, were going through various stages of transformation including redundancy and when previously, I would have had exemplary 1-2-1's with my director, things had started to slip, and my performance was not as great as my track record. I started to struggle, I was trying to be all things to everyone and neglected my own self-care.

Most days, I would go home exhausted and the easiest thing for me to do was to order a takeaway for me and the kids and fall into bed completely worn out. So, you can see why I became morbidly obese. My diet was not sustaining me in a healthy way.

My head and brain were constantly working on overdrive, I was worried about losing my job and the security and purpose it gave me. My body and brain were in a constant state of alert, something that I now know is called "Fight or Flight mode". My emotional state was under constant attack. Often feeling worried and anxious about my mom, my job and whether I was being the mom I wanted to be for my kids.

> **Fight or flight refers to a physiological reaction that occurs when we are in the presence of something that is mentally or physically terrifying. It is triggered by a release of hormones that prepare your body to either stay and deal with the threat or to flee and escape. It was my body's way of dealing with all the built-up stress I was encountering.**

My body was reacting to my autonomic nervous system. It was affecting my heart rate and my respiratory rate; I was experiencing panic attacks every time I left the house. I had huge amounts of paranoia, I felt everyone was judging me and looking at me and so I began to lock myself away whenever I could.

I felt safer at home than being out. All the usual social activities that I had previously taken part in came to a grinding halt. I basically isolated myself from the world.

My digestive system was in poor health, I often had bouts of IBS that were probably not helped by my poor diet.

> **IBS (irritable bowel syndrome) is a chronic gastrointestinal disorder that affects the large intestine causing diarrhea, abdominal pain, cramps, bloating and flatulence.**
> **There is no known cure but medication and improving your diet can help to ease the symptoms.**
> **More common in females, it can be intermittent or last several years, even sometimes whole life.**

Over time my general mental and physical health continued to decline. I had become disengaged with my new husband; my libido was affected, and I started to question everything he said or did.

My paranoia grew. I felt that everyone was conspiring against me. I lost trust in humanity. If you could not trust your husband or your kids, the very people that you loved and thought the most of, what was there left?

It was a sad time in my life. I did not feel I could speak to him because I thought it would result in an argument or I would feel even more loathing. Everything felt like it was a negative, even though I was fighting hard to see the positive. It was a vicious cycle.

> **The autonomic nervous system is the primary mechanism in control of the fight-or-flight response and its role is mediated by two different components: the sympathetic nervous system and the parasympathetic nervous system. Before I get too scientific, the easiest way to describe it was that it was affecting my adrenal gland. This gland affects your blood pressure, blood sugar and your immune system. This was the science behind how I was feeling and why I was feeling so low.**

I was in a constant spiral of low mood, fatigue, and hopelessness. Normal everyday functions were becoming more and more difficult. This was not an overnight mental health issue; it was a build-up of struggles for nearly a year.

Due to my ongoing poor health I decided to leave my job at the end of 2013. This was a massive decision for me and not one that I came to overnight, because I loved the variation of my housing role, the teams I worked with and the opportunity to learn something new every day.

For approximately 6 months before I made the decision to leave, I got up every morning and arrived at work, thinking today was going to be a better day and yet the stress just got too much. I could not cope with my role.

For years, I had been given numerous opportunities to have promotions with every appraisal being extremely positive, I was finding that **my appraisals were now filled with negativity, I was missing milestones, and my teams and my work quality was suffering**.

I eventually concluded that I had no alternative but to leave. I thought that my teams would be better off without me at the helm.

It was not an easy decision to reach because I was the breadwinner, my salary was double that of my husband. I knew that my lifestyle would have to change drastically, I tried to remain optimistic and thought that I would be able to find another job easily.

Unfortunately, other job opportunities did not materialise as I had expected and so began months of my mental health spiralling downwards to the point when I was seriously contemplating ending it all and taking my own life.

I would spend most of my day in bed, not showering or taking care of my diet. My normal everyday routine was out the window.

After months of this, I was jolted back to reality when my son asked me to go on a walk with him. I was reluctant to move but eventually I dragged myself out of bed and got dressed.

My appearance was like a shadow of my former self. **My hair was dishevelled, I had lost interest in applying makeup and I just put on any outfit that I felt comfortable in**, usually joggers and a baggy top.

As we walked in our beautiful country park. I was not aware of my surroundings. I was just totally consumed in my own dark world. I'm not sure why but suddenly I felt that I needed to open up to my son about how I was feeling.

He was only 18yrs old, and I was in too deep a state of misery to even begin to question whether I should talk to him and burden him with my worries. He was there and I needed someone to speak to.

I thought that he could understand why I was feeling like I was, after all, he had been with me throughout my journey, he knew about my struggles with my mom's terminal illness and what I had gone through in my career.

I told him that **I felt hopeless and that I had given up on life and that I wanted to end it all**, for their sake as well as mine. It was the most difficult conversation of my life and looking back my son was not the person that I should have had this conversation with. I was the mom, the matriarch, the one that had been strong and kept us together through all our life challenges.

Like, when my first marriage broke down and I left our family home with my three young children. I was on a low salary and only working part time, so the best option we had was to find a rental property. Over the following year, we moved from rental property to rental property.

The first rental property was perfect. Just around the corner from my kids' school and their friends, had 3 bedrooms and was in a good state of repair with a long garden, suitable for my kids to play in.

After 6 months, we found out unexpectedly that the landlady wanted her property back after her relationship had broken down. The timing was not great because it was just before Christmas. So, I needed to act swiftly. The best available rental property I could find, that was nearest to my kids' school, was a 2-bed terrace property, which was a short drive away.

I felt that I had to take it. It was the best option we had. I thought that as soon as I could find another property closer to my kids' school we could move again. We moved in and I did my best to make the Christmas as best as I could. It was not ideal, because I was sleeping on the sofa and had no space of my own, however my main concern was to make sure my kids were ok.

Just a few weeks into the New Year a property came up on the estate where we had lived previously. Perfect! The kids would be back where their friends were, and they would be able to walk to school again. The landlord had moved abroad, so it looked like we had a prospect of a long term let or hopefully an opportunity to plant roots for a few years. This would give me time to find a full-time job and start saving to get a deposit and explore my house buying options.

Once again, our plans had to change as after a few months they had decided that living abroad was not for them and they wanted to move back home. We were back looking for a new home again.

I was then told about another house on the estate that was going to be coming on the market. Brilliant, I knew the landlord and was aware that they rented properties with a view to it being a longer term let. The condition was not great, although I had got some money from my finance settlement in my divorce that I could use to redecorate and carpet, just like I had done with each of the other properties.

I could make it into home, and I decided to invest my money into doing up the property because it was hopefully going to be long term. Or that was my hope at the time.

Back to the conversation with my son, I cannot recall what was said that day, but something just clicked in my head. Some people call it a light bulb moment and it must have been because I suddenly realised what was important in my life. My kids.

I wanted to be here to see my children grow up into their adulthood. I believed I could find a purpose again and I knew that there was so much more I wanted to achieve in life. **I had turned a massive corner and decided to take responsibility for my own health and wellbeing**.

I knew I needed help, so I reached out to find the right support. If I were going to transform my life, habits and improve my interpersonal skills and mindset, I could not do it alone. I also recognised that I had a passion for helping others and decided to explore how I could do that in my new brave world.

Over the course of the next year I grew stronger, investing in transforming my life for the better. I began to eat a healthier diet and took up cycling. I prioritised my own self-care and decided to start studying and learning more about personal development and interpersonal skills topics.

At first, I found the transformation challenging, but I chose to **focus on the positives** and when I saw improvements however big or small, I knew that I was making progress, and that spurred me on.

I began to plan my meals, I made positive choices, eating more fruit and vegetables, and alternated between meat and plant-based food. I joined weight watchers and went to be weighed each week and when I saw that my weight and dress size improved, this helped me to stick with it.

Cycling was a massive help too. At first, I would cycle locally around the block, starting off with short rides and then week on week, I would increase my mileage.

Creating a positive routine, to prioritise cycling into my life was a massive bonus. Every Sunday, I dedicated the day to cycling and I continue to do this to this day. Over the last few years, my recovery rate has improved, and I have completed several bike tours, with my biggest ride being from Worcestershire to Cornwall completely independently. I covered over 500 miles, with all my gear and I pitched my tent along the way.

I was so proud of my achievement, and I managed to raise funds for the Charity; British Heart Foundation, a charity close to my heart because my Grandad passed away due to a heart attack. I also used my cycling as a mindfulness tool, using every opportunity to take in the sights and sounds of my journeys, using all my senses.

I came up with the idea to start my own business after months of being unsuccessful in finding employment. I thought that my experiences and life transformations could help others.

It was ***my way of giving back to others based on the overwhelming help that I had received***. I wanted to give others the tools and techniques to prevent the same things happening to them and to help them have the skills they need to thrive. I knew I had a lot to learn about running a business because I had always been employed by large corporate organisations. The skill set needed to run your own business is completely different to being employed.

I enrolled on several courses, about running your own business as well as ILM (Institute of Leadership) courses. It was after spending a year on my new business that I then took the step to become a mature student and enrol at university and complete an Entrepreneurship Degree.

My Business evolved and diversified, I rebranded and changed my focus to look at offering training, which was the right decision. It was once I did this that I found that it was building an audience and getting recognised.

My mission statement and business objectives were now aligned to my personal goals. **It was completely the right thing to do**. Starting your own business is a long process and not all businesses have overnight success, it takes perseverance, resilience, and commitment, and is a bit like a rollercoaster ride, however I knew that it was the right decision for me at this stage in my life.

My destiny was in my hands, I was totally responsible for every decision I made and that felt good.

It is important to say that there are a range of services out there if you currently experience any of the symptoms that I did. I remember speaking to the Samaritans when I was at my lowest ebb. That phone call helped me hugely. Having someone to listen to my concerns and anxieties at that time without having to burden my family and without judgement was just what

I needed. I also attended some community meetings with the charity MIND.

This helped me step back out into society, relaxed my mind, and helped me with coping strategies when I felt a panic attack coming on. There are a range of people that can help you and these are just two of the charities that helped me. It is okay to ask for help, you are not alone.

You just need to take that step and ask.

'No Such Thing As Normal', is a great book on all things Mental Health by Bryony Gordon.

Today's Environment

Well, who would have thought it, the pandemic has been a time like no other? **The world has been turned upside down** with everyone's life being affected in one way or another by COVID and Lockdown.

Some positively but for many it has had a huge impact on their mental health.

People's mental health is strongly associated with social and economic circumstances like concerns over health, worries about employment, job security and unemployment and your housing situation.

This is something that I can very much relate to after having to move 4 times in one year. Your home is your sanctuary and a place where you feel safe. It has a massive impact on your Wellbeing.

You can certainly understand why so many people are struggling now and are experiencing anxiety and stress, especially as many industries have been so negatively impacted by the pandemic.

The reality is the security of your job, health and home are all being affected. I totally get it and mix that with other social factors like digital transformation, concerns over our planet and our health care system namely the NHS, it is no wonder that anxieties are reaching fever pitch for so many.

It is what makes us human, and you can take a certain amount of comfort from the fact that we are all in this together. You cannot turn on a TV screen, listen to a podcast or read an article that does not in some way refer to mental health and people's wellbeing in some shape or form.

The best piece of advice I can give at this point is to say; You are not alone, you and thousands like you, are going through these same worries and concerns.

When I think of how I am now thriving and how I would have coped, had I not invested a serious amount of time into my own personal development, well, it does not bear thinking about.

Different groups have been adversely affected, with those on lower incomes, younger people, people with children and people that have a diagnosed mental health illness, having higher levels of anxiety and depression.

Social isolation and the feeling of loneliness has had a particular impact on people who live alone and with underlying health conditions. The reality is that many people only left their homes for essential tasks because of fears for their safety.

**Emerging evidence on COVID 19's impact on people's mental health demonstrates that two thirds of adults are somewhat or very worried about how COVID 19 will affect their lives moving forward (L,Marshall. 2020).
The most common themes are worries for their future, feelings of stress & anxiety and boredom brought on by furlough and loss of employment.**

Whether you suffer from a mental health condition or not, the point is here people's confidence has been affected which has resulted in a change in the way we live our lives.

**Having positive mental health is strongly associated today with a healthy diet and good physical health. Historically, mental health and physical health have been largely treated separately. Following a vast amount of research by academics, this thought process has been flipped on its head. People with higher levels of distress and worries are more likely to have increased risks of coronary heart disease and are 32% more likely to die from a cancerous illness. Lifestyle factors such as taking exercise can release feel good chemicals in the brain called endorphins.
You can find out more via the British Heart Foundation website:**

https://www.bhf.org.uk/informationsupport

Burnout to BOLD

Worsening mental health can be affected by many different drivers such as social isolation, job and financial losses, housing insecurity, loss of support mechanisms, if you worked on the front line and reduced access to mental health services.

I appreciate that for some people, taking up a sport may feel like a big ask. I recall when the doctor diagnosed, that I was morbidly obese, I was a dress size 22. I knew that I had to make dramatic changes to my lifestyle but the thought of joining a sports club, gym or sport event filled me with dread.

This was linked to my feelings of self-worth and self-esteem and was all connected to my mindset and poor mental health. The point here is that short bursts of 10 minutes of brisk walking can have huge benefits to your mood, energy levels and mental alertness. Everyone can start somewhere.

According to the Mental Health Foundation report, it is recommended that an average adult should take part in between 75 and 150 mins of exercise per week. When you break this down, it equates to just over 20 mins per day. That is more achievable, I believe. Physical activity can be amazingly effective in relieving stress. Higher active people tend to have lower stress rates, than people who are inactive.

You can find out more via the Mental Health Foundation website:

https://www.mentalhealth.org.uk/publications/how-to-using-exercise

I took up cycling. Starting with a leisurely cycle around my neighbourhood. I continued to build this up every week and when I started to notice the differences both physically and mentally, it gave me the motivation and determination to continue to invest in my physical wellbeing and massively helped my mood.

Reassessing your Priorities

One of the positives to have emerged from the pandemic is that it has led people and society to reassess their priorities. It has given us the opportunity to rethink what is important to us, move away from autopilot and concentrate more on our own sense of wellbeing. This includes self-care in all its various forms both physically, mentally, and socially.

Historically, pandemics of this nature resulted in changes to our society. The biggest concern we are now facing is about social inequalities. That is where I believe things like self-responsibility and accountability come in. It is easy to blame others when things go wrong in our lives, however we live in a knowledge society with so many things at our fingertips. **Our destinies are for us to decide**. Now is a great time to reflect and decide our path.

That is what I had to do when I was on the brink of ending my life. I got to a crossroads, was I going to sink into a deeper sense of poor mental health or was I going to take responsibility and turn things around?

Thankfully, I took the latter decision. I just had to work out how I was going to do it, what my purpose was, where were my passions, and what did I want from life?

This is now your opportunity to reset your priorities and reinvent what you want out of life.

You will have short term goals or maybe like me you might want to transform your life for the better. Take a change in career, start up your own business, change how and when you want to work. Have you heard about the gig economy revolution? The gig economy is higher risk, but it can certainly give you better life choices, you work when you want, with who you want pretty much.

It is like the emergence of Agile working. It gives you an opportunity to work how and when you want, giving you the opportunity to look at your strengths and interests and basically start an enterprise from there.

Maybe your goal is to be able to take your kids to school and pick them up every day. By having your own business, you can work the hours you want. Or say you want to get that home versus life balance back and only work 4 days a week on your terms. Self-employment gives you these types of opportunities.

Okay, it is not without risks, and you will need to consider things like your financial commitments, but the benefits, in my experience, far outweigh the negatives.

You **will** need to be self-motivated to do this, and you will need to get yourself out there and build a network. That is **why it is important to find your passion** because once you do, you will find the motivation that gets you up in the morning.

On a personal level, I went from earning a great salary in the corporate world to having a few years of building up my customer base with a low income, but it helped me plan better. I have become savvier with what I spend my money on, better at managing my time and better at organising my life.

That has got to be a good thing, right? This way I can redirect my income into doing more of the things I love to do. Like cycling and going on adventures and exploring some of the lovely places our country has to offer. That gives me better life choices and is hugely beneficial to my own health and wellbeing.

I appreciate for some of you, this may not be the right time but then I ask you, **if not now, when?** Use this time to give yourself a fresh start, if only by investing in your own health and wellbeing, taking responsibility for your mental health, and moving forward positively.

Things you could explore further.

After I reached the crossroads when I was at my lowest, the only way I could go was up. The rest of the chapters in this book will plot out the different paths that I took to get me to where I am today. I appreciate that everyone is different and what worked for me may not work for you, but I am sure there will be something you can take from my various personal development twists and turns.

As a result of my poor mental health, I locked myself away. I cut off from everyone, friends, family, work colleagues the lot. My first step was to start learning to trust again, make new friends, and start functioning like a member of society. It was at this point I learnt about MIND, the mental health charity.

> https://www.mind.org.uk/

Again, it was about taking responsibility for my own wellbeing. I started to look out for myself, and I found the help I needed.

MIND is a mental health charity that helps individuals and carers get the support and respect they need to aid recovery from a mental health illness. I was fortunate that I found a group local to where I live that ran a programme to help us socialise.

If you need help, then reach out to MIND and find out what support is available local to you. This is where I first learnt about using Mindfulness, something that I am a great advocate for. I will cover this in my next chapter.

It was around this time that I also accepted that I needed to do something to help improve my physical wellbeing such as my diet. Remember I was morbidly obese and take-aways were a way of life rather than a treat. Especially, after spending months hiding away, lying in bed, not dressing, washing, or taking exercise.

I learnt about the **5 Ways to Wellbeing** model that the Government had developed in 2008. The whole premise of this initiative was to try and develop a model that could help people improve their whole health and wellbeing, decrease mental health problems in a holistic way.

This for me was and still is the best thing that I did in my recovery, and I completely swear by it, it works, 100% if you are committed to making a positive change and take responsibility and remain consistent. It gave me structure, focus and most importantly, it gave me the tools I needed to move forward.

It is funny because in my third chapter I look at confidence and self-esteem and while the **5 Ways to**

Wellbeing helped me with my confidence, conversely, the more I learnt about self-esteem, self-worth, and confidence the better I began to feel about myself and gained motivation to remain committed to it.

This was not a straight path to my life transformation; it was really a weaving path of learning and discovery. Various topics and initiatives coming together and complimenting each other in different ways.
Remember, it is the result that counts.

Resilience is something that was a hot topic of conversation especially after the year of lockdowns back in 2020. It really was the year the world came to a halt, and it really tested most people's resilience.

There are lots of experts emerging in this field, many of whom I have learnt much about resilience from. I want to give you my spin on what it means to me and how it made a difference in my life, and I will share that with you, what I have learnt along my journey.

The great thing about resilience is that it can be built on as you move forward in life, your levels of resilience would have been built from the moment you were born. However, your family environment, your childhood experiences, and your values and beliefs will all influence how resilient you are at various stages in your life.

I will dig further into this topic and share my different experiences that shaped my resilience within my ditty at the end of my Resilience chapter.

Emotional intelligence, also known as **EI**, is a topic I cover in this book and to be honest, it has only been within the last 8 years of my life that I have fully understood what this is, but on reflection I have been using **EI** throughout my life.

It was when I sat down and read the book **'Emotional Intelligence 2.0'**, by Jean Greaves and Travis Bradberry, while holidaying in Cyprus, that I had that light bulb moment. Ah-ha, that is what **EI** is and how it can help you get on in life!

It is something that can be built upon throughout life and I would highly recommend you start with reading the book. I think it is a game changer in life to learn more about this topic simply because it can have such a gigantic impact on yourself and with the relationships you have.

Are leaders made or born? I have read numerous research articles and books about this topic. You can look back at leaders in history and their background and form your own opinions.

For me leadership is something that anyone can do, I do not say that flippantly. It takes a lifetime of continual learning, self-belief, empathy, and the right kind of mindset to be a great historic leader. Anyone at any age, gender or diversity can lead. Great leaders often have similar characteristics.

Have a look at the book **'7 Habits of Highly Effective People'**, by Stephen Covey, it is an easy read and is an excellent self-help book, if you aspire to lead in your career or life. Did I ever believe that I was a leader? Well, I will explore this topic further within this book and hopefully inspire you to lead too.

Everyone is unique and when it comes to leadership, it is about getting the right person for the job. Based on knowledge, skills, and experience. I will talk you through my leadership journey in the book. It has been a bumpy ride, but it all adds to the richness of my life, and it certainly can build your character, hopefully for the better.

Change is one thing that we can guarantee in life, who starts their careers with a road map for the rest of their lives? Well, seriously no-one. You may have career aspirations, goals, and certain interests that you are passionate about that can shape your direction, but **the reality is anything can happen**. That is why I want to explore 'Managing Change' within this book because it is how you approach change that will shape your future successes.

My world was turned upside down after my mental health illness and if you had met me prior to my illness, you would have never thought in a million years that I could have been that person that retreated to my bed and stayed there for 6 months. In fact, I found it hard to believe it myself.

My recovery did not happen overnight. It has taken years of personal development and using reflection to appreciate that I had a lot to learn. I have come out of it a stronger and hopefully a better person for my journey. This is where responsibility, positivity and accountability come in.

It might be that this chapter helps you to discover what area of personal development you need to explore further and feel free to jump ahead if you do have that clarity. I am just sharing with you the different interpersonal skills topics that helped me learn more about myself, my strengths, weaknesses and ultimately helped me transform my life for the better.

Burnout to BOLD

My Ditty: The day my wellies saved me

"Come on Chels, are you ready yet?" I was screaming at the top of my lungs up the stairs. I had literally only been up for about 15 minutes myself, yes, my hair was brushed, but I have not put any makeup on. My usual routine would be to slap on some eyeliner and mascara and straighten my blonde hair. Not today though, "Chelsie!", I screamed again, "We need to be there in half an hour!".

I was filled with nerves and my stomach felt in knots, because I was taking my beautiful first daughter for an operation and whilst it was a routine operation, I also understood that any operation comes with some risks. I shouted up the stairs for the final time, "Chels, I am going to wait in the car!", I then rushed out of the door and sat in my car with the engine humming.

I sat there exhausted, and the day had only just begun, Chelsie jumped into the car and before she had time to put on her seatbelt, I was reversing off the drive. We then started the drive into Birmingham City Centre. We had only got halfway, and I could feel my stomach start to bubble and gurgle.

At this point I was morbidly obese and had a poor diet, and for the last 2 years I had irritable bowel syndrome. While this was not diagnosed, I knew in my heart of hearts it was partly due to my diet of takeaways and fatty foods.

My staple foods were a chocolate bar, biscuits, and cakes. Pretty much anything that I could eat on the go.

Burnout to BOLD

"Oh, Chels, I need the loo". Chelsie started to laugh, "What are you going to do?", she said. "I don't know, I guess I will have to try and hold on until we get to Birmingham's Children's Hospital, there will be a toilet in the reception area, I'm sure'. The rest of the journey was spent in almost silence while I was concentrating on trying to get my stomach in order, while we did have some elements of small talk; mainly about how she was feeling about the operation, in part I was focused on getting there and finding a toilet.

We had just started to see the giant skyscrapers as we drove up the Bristol Road into the outskirts of the City Centre. "Okay, Chels, can you look at the Sat Nav and find us the closest car park to the Children's", I said. We then followed the myriad of roads around the ring road of Birmingham, until we came across the NCP.

The whole time, my stomach continued to cramp, and I was desperate to find a loo. I drove around the car park looking to find a suitable place to park up. "Oh, NO!", I said. "What is it?" said Chelsie. 'I need to go to the loo!', 'It's okay we are nearly there' she said. "You don't understand, I need to go to the loo and need to go now!!"." Mom, what are you going to do? You'll have to wait!".

I was driving around each level and all the cars parked up, were lined up in a row and there were people milling around returning to their cars and getting their car park tickets. "I need to find a quieter spot to park up, Chels", I am going to have to go now!". I then pulled up into a quieter parking space in the corner of the Car Park.

I then jumped out of the car and opened the boot. What did I have that I could use to help me? I then saw my Wedding Wellies that I had kept in the boot of my car.

"This will do", I said to Chelsie. "Mom, what are you doing with them, Wellies?". The shock and disgust were written all over her face. "Surely, you can wait, we are nearly there?", she said. "I am sorry, I need to go, and I need to go now!". I had become numb to the embarrassment of having to dash to the toilet at a moment's notice because I had become used to the symptoms of IBS.

"You go get the parking ticket", I said. I then clambered into the rear of the car with my wedding wellie in hand and I guess you can imagine what happened next. Poor Chelsie was mortified, and she giggled with embarrassment at the same time.

The whole start of the day was a blur of rushing around and panic. Not a great way to start what was a monumental day for my daughter. I stepped out of the car with the Wedding Wellie in my hand. I had a huge sense of relief; my stomach cramps had subsided, and I felt that I could now concentrate on what was going to be a long day ahead.

We then walked down the spiral of concrete stairs and I still had the wellie in my hand and as we entered on to the street, there was a euro bin that I could put the wellie into. We both then walked across to the huge entrance of the hospital, laughing about the events of our journey to that point.

The rest of the day was completely textbook, Chelsie had her operation to remove her tonsils successfully and she was able to come home that very evening.

Back at home we retold the stories of the day and laughed about the turbulent start, and while it was filled with humour, the serious part of this story was about my own health and wellbeing and state of mind.

I have since retold this story numerous times and recalled how my Wellies had saved me that day, however the reality is that it has serious undertones about my mental health and how I was chaotic and in poor health.

Since changing my diet radically, I no longer have IBS; thankfully, and while, the story of how my wellie had saved me that day is just a distant memory, albeit funny in nature, it is a stark reminder of one episode in my poor mental health period.

Burnout to BOLD

Burnout to BOLD

CHAPTER 2: 5 WAYS TO WELLBEING

This model is, as I said in Chapter 1, is something that the Government office for science developed in collaboration with the New Economics Foundation (NEF) in 2008.

> https://www.gov.uk/government/publications/five-ways-to-mental-wellbeing

The whole premise of this initiative was to try and develop a model that could help people to improve their whole health and wellbeing whilst decreasing mental health problems in a holistic way. There is so much evidence to suggest the positive benefits to our mental health by being healthier and physically active.

I am going to walk you through the 5 Ways to Wellbeing model and share with you my stories of how this model has helped to transform my life.

- ♥ Be Active
- ♥ Keep Learning
- ♥ Connect
- ♥ Take notice!
- ♥ Give

Be Active

This is exactly what it says on the tin. We can easily become complacent about our physical health, especially in recent times when we have been predominantly working and living our day to day lives in and around the home. **It is hugely important to take some form of physical activity daily.**

Whilst it's obvious that being physically healthier will improve your life expectancy, it is important to ensure you maintain physical health whatever your level of ability. Obvious yes, but how many of us actually do it?

Whatever your preference; walking, cycling, something more extreme; it is important to make time to be active. From half an hour a day, working out at home to a YouTube fitness video, to taking part in a weekly local community park run.

The point here is that you need to ensure you make time within your weekly schedule to do something. To **create ongoing and positive activity habits**.

I remember when I first started using this model, the thought of any kind of physical activity seemed daunting to me because I was overweight and totally unfit.

Everyone can start making progress.

I got a puppy back in 2014 and whilst I am not advocating that you rush out and buy a dog (this type of investment takes a lot of commitment and thought) for us it was the best decision we ever made. This was the very first step to changing my direction for the better and incorporating physical activity every day.

Every morning when we got up the first thing we would do, after having our early morning cuppa, would be to take Bourbon, our springer spaniel, for a walk to the local park. It was a great first step to moving towards a healthier lifestyle. Baby steps.

Everyone who knows me knows that I am now a keen

cyclist and I love to do Bike Tours.

This involves plotting a journey and taking everything with us for the trip, sometimes for a weekend or maybe for weeks at a time. I can do this now because my body has been trained to do it, but at the start the thought of cycling even just around the block filled me with dread.

Your body is like a fine oiled machine, the more you do something the better you become.

I did struggle initially, finding little joy in cycling at first, but then, quite quickly in fact, I noticed that my breathing and recovery rates were improving, and the most important thing was that I was enjoying it.

I was getting a buzz out of being able to go further and felt great at the end of the ride. My strength and capacity built up over time and now we dedicate every Sunday to cycling whatever the weather.

The other thing I started doing was Yoga classes, which moved to online classes during lockdown with Anna Curnow Yoga. This helped with my flexibility and focus as well as being massively useful for mindfulness.

These are now **my** passions. I appreciate that for you it could be something else. Find something you enjoy, and you want to do more and more.

It is a bit like when you are building a snowman, it gains momentum. This along with healthy eating is a winning combination. I will write more about this later in the take notice section.

Why not try several different activities out first discover what you enjoy and works best for you?

Keep Learning

What is your approach to personal development? Have you been in the same job role for several years and are happy being in your comfort zone, doing the same things day in and day out? What if I told you that you have so much more untapped potential? What if you stretched out of your comfort zone and learnt a new skill or new role, something that gives you purpose, something that ignites your passions?

That was me, I lived in my comfort zone in my role as a Head of Service in a Housing Association. Yes, I would attend any training that could help me improve the services I was responsible for but was I achieving my full potential? Maybe not, or maybe so, but due to my poor mental health, I hit a crossroads.

After my recovery, I decided to start my own enterprise. This was me moving out of my comfort zone and into my stretch zone. I had a great vision of what I wanted to achieve by having my own business; autonomy, home versus work life balance and the opportunity to have a robust personal development plan and ultimately achieving my full potential.

I started my first business with the aim of **helping others to improve their wellbeing**. Over the course of the next year, I realised that I did not have all the skills and knowledge necessary to make it a successful business. So, I took a huge leap of faith and began to explore the possibility of going to university to do a degree in Business.

I left school with poor GCSE grades. I must take responsibility for this because my focus in those days was to have fun with my friends and I was more interested in taking part in team sports and PE. Does this sound like you?

With a fresh focus and years of work experience behind me, I knew that if I had **the right mindset and focus**, I could progress and achieve a degree. The thought of doing this filled me with dread. What if I was not bright enough? What if I could not keep up with the pace of learning? Would I understand academic speak and the jargon that is used in this type of establishment?

We often stick with what we know, and it was only after I read the book '**The Chimp Paradox'**, by Prof Steve Peters, that I began to understand that I was responsible for my own self-sabotage.

Your mindset and your view of what you can achieve is the only thing that holds you back. The book was a revelation. It is a mind management program that can help you achieve success, confidence, and happiness. This is something that we all want to achieve in life, right?

Here is where I ask you to take a good look at your life. Are you fulfilled in your life, are you enjoying your job, do you experience everything that you want to do? If the answer is yes, then fantastic you do not need my help.

If you answered no, well then, I urge you to read on. Start by writing down your dreams. Then let us work back from there. As part of this 5 Ways to Wellbeing chapter, I have a handout that can help you.

Visit our website for our FREE '5 Ways to Wellbeing' downloadable booklet:

Our website is
www.advanceyourwellbeing.co.uk

It could be that you, like me, decide to return to learning and become a mature student or maybe something simpler, like an online course. The point here is to develop a robust personal development plan and start working towards your goals.

You can achieve your dreams, you just need commitment, dedication, and laser focus.

My Dreams – *list your dreams here:*

_____
_____
_____
_____
_____
_____
_____
_____
_____
_____
_____
_____
_____
_____
_____
_____

Connect

Humans are sociable creatures and, in a world, where Mental Health is a growing concern, it is even more important for us to build relationships and prevent feelings of isolation. This is something that can massively help our wellbeing. I read an interesting article; **Loneliness, Isolation and Social Support Factors**, (L, Saltzman et al) that explains this in more detail.

It explains how in a time of crisis, social support is emphasized as a coping mechanism. It makes perfect sense. After I spent months locking myself away from the world, cutting myself off from my family and friends, I began to understand the importance of these relationships and how by isolating myself, I was doing more harm than good.

I then started building my network up again bit by bit. The impact of this was a revelation and helped me build trust again, something that I had lost but wanted back. The other positive side to this was that my confidence began to build again.

During this time, I did a lot of self-reflection and I learnt what my strengths and weaknesses were, (although I prefer to call weaknesses 'opportunities to grow'). I had a growing feeling of self-worth. I discovered and felt that I could make a positive impact on others, with what I had learnt on my wellbeing journey & recovery from poor mental health.

To some reading this, it may sound a bit melodramatic but if you have found yourself in the same head space that I was in, you will completely get where I am coming from. I was moving away from feelings of despair and pity, from catastrophising every event, to a more positive outlook on all aspects of my life. This all came out of **being with and around other positive people**.

That is when I had another light bulb moment and decided that I could find my purpose again and that is where my business idea first started to take shape. I looked around at other businesswomen and thought, surely if they can do it, then I am sure I could too.

At that time, I was not entirely sure of how my business was going to work, I just knew that I wanted to help others and try to give people the tools and help that could prevent the spiral of poor mental health, and more positively help individuals thrive and achieve their full potential.

I spent the first year of running my own business learning from others and this is my mantra for life, you can always learn something new every day. To do this, you need to connect with others.

One of the positives that has come out of the recent pandemic is that most of us have increased our confidence in using more technology, this has resulted in us being able to connect with anyone, anywhere in the world.

Building relationships and networking can help you in so many ways but the biggest thing I would say I have learnt from my experience, is the positive impacts that people have on your health & wellbeing, your personal growth and on your ability to succeed.

It is incredibly important to understand the impact that your relationships have on your life i.e., do they have a positive impact, do they spur you on to achieve your goals, do they create an environment that nurtures personal growth?

These were all questions that I asked myself as I re-emerged into the world and especially when I started my own business. I wanted to surround myself with positive can-do attitudes and with people that did not judge or those 'Never Nellies'. You know the ones, they are the people that put obstacles in the way of everything, always offering a reason as to why something will not be a success or are just 'woe is me'.

The reality is that you *will* come across these people in your life, that is just the way things are, but the great thing here, is that **you get to choose**, you get to choose as to whether you invest your time into these 'Never Nellies' or whether you walk away and surround yourself with the right kind of people.

Take Notice

How often do you wake up in the morning and just go on autopilot, doing your usual routine without using the opportunity to see the joy in all things in life no matter how small? Be it choosing an outfit that helps you to feel great, enjoying your breakfast, or just the joy of sipping on your first cuppa of the day.

It is all about being mindful and we explore this further in this book.

Life is not a dress rehearsal, you may only be here once, so how about making it count, living the life of your dreams and ultimately achieving your full potential?

Okay, so this may seem flippant, but the point I want to stress here is about taking notice, it is about being grateful for all the little things in life and just **living in the present moment**. A lot of people refer to 'taking notice' as 'mindfulness', and it is but mindfulness is so much more than that.

Burnout to BOLD

Quite often in life we get consumed with worrying about things that are out of our control or have feelings of anxiety for fear of the unknown. The reality is we are putting ourselves into a negative mindset, which is counterproductive to our wellbeing, or as some people call it, 'self-sabotage'.

Let me take you back to 2013, this was when I was working in a corporate environment, trying to be all things to all people. My mom needed support because she had COPD and I was trying my best to help her while juggling work commitments which were ever evolving and my role as a mom to three wonderful kids.

I was struggling with all the commitments that I had, and self-care was something I never practised. When I got home from work each evening, exhausted, I would choose the easy option and order take-aways or eat quick and easy processed foods.

Now looking back, I completely understand how my weight had escalated to the point where I had been diagnosed as morbidly obese. I was the heaviest I have ever been. I was in a dress size 22. What fuel I was giving my body was not the best and I was just eating all the wrong things rather than making positive diet choices.

Fast forward to today and I have totally transformed my approach towards what I eat, and mealtime is a totally different affair. I have learnt how to cook healthier meals with fresh ingredients, I take time to enjoy and taste my meals.

During lockdown I also started to bake, like lots of

people out there and yes banana bread is one of the cakes I made many times. That is another new skill to add to my list.

This has all resulted in me maintaining my current weight and dress size and having treats in moderation. Although if I am honest, I did put on a few lockdown pounds. Hey, I am human after all.

The relevance here is about; **Taking Notice**, especially about what we are putting into our bodies and slowing down and taking the time to taste and enjoy your meals.

I am a huge fan of using spices and herbs in my cooking now because it can help things taste so much better. I always plan my week's meals before I do my weekly shop, that way I know I am getting a balanced diet.

It is nothing scientific, I have a notebook, where I compile a menu for the week and then on the opposite page, I write my shopping list. The other bonus of this, is that I am only spending what I need to, rather than impulse buying, and reducing my food waste.

To help with my weight loss I took up cycling as you already know, and as well as the physical benefits of cycling, it's my opportunity to practice mindfulness and 'Take Notice'.

I use it as a time to practice self-care, relax and just appreciate what is around me, like the changing of the seasons or enjoying the stunning scenery that I find myself in. **It is a form of meditation for me**. It certainly helps me top up my Wellbeing tank both physically and mentally.

Give

Quite often in life we can get consumed with our own lives and caught up with what we do not have or focus on negatives but let me flip this on its head. What if we **take the time to think about the positive things we have**?

Your health, your family & friends, the roof above your head. If we all just spent more time thinking about how fortunate we all really are, then it could have a massive impact on your Wellbeing.

Sometimes it takes stepping out of your own bubble to appreciate what others are facing and appreciating what we have and being more grateful for our own lives. For this element of the **5 Ways to Wellbeing**, I decided to do some volunteering and I continue to do volunteering to this day and hope to continue in the future.

Through networking, I found out about a homeless charity that did outreach in the streets and I would go out on a Sunday evening and provide food and hot drinks along with items of clothing to help those who found themselves living in shop doorways. What an incredibly humbling experience.

I also did a sleep out with my family for the night in November a few years ago now for Framework in Nottingham which helped me appreciate the warmth of sleeping in my lovely home, this helped to raise money for those less fortunate than myself and it certainly was a cold night and made me realise that doing that night after night would not be conducive for your health and wellbeing and made me realise how lucky I was to have a place to lay my head with the benefits of heating and hot water.

These are things in life we can all take for granted. I then started to volunteer with a local food bank called Foodbank Birmingham and we would make a scrummy 3 course meal for the local community. It was amazing to see the people that we had coming through the doors, professional people that had found themselves out of work through redundancy and families on low incomes that were struggling to feed their children. It certainly helped to open my eyes to the benefits that these food banks bring to their local communities.

I now volunteer with two different organisations that fit in with my current lifestyle of being a self-employed woman. I appreciate with the busyness of life and especially for those people that are employed full-time finding the time to volunteer could be a daunting prospect, how could you fit it all in?

I would say this is an opportunity to be creative. I walk my dog Bourbon most mornings and while walking I do a litter pick in my local park. It takes me the same amount of time and if everyone did just a little bit it has a big impact. It does not have to take you from doing what you love in your spare time, it's just about shifting your mindset and giving back in a way that fits your lifestyle.

Another example could be that you enjoy taking part in your local park run each week, and perhaps one of these weeks you could volunteer to be a marshal? The possibilities are endless.

Many businesses are looking at their ethical strategies and as such have developed Corporate Social Responsibility policies. What does this mean, well for one of my volunteering opportunities I am an Enterprise Advisor with the Careers & Enterprise Company.

> **https://www.careersandenterprise.co.uk/**

The role involves me supporting schools' careers leads and bringing pupils and businesses together to enrich careers choices for young people. The hope is that it will inspire pupils to consider other careers roles and I totally enjoy the creativity that comes from pupils.

The other bonus for me is that it enables me to network with my potential future customers and build relationships. It is a win-win situation for mutual benefit.

Visit their website to find out how you can get involved, this is a nationwide initiative, and you will find there are plenty of ways you can get involved with your local schools.

The other volunteer role I do is with Extracare Charitable Trust. This is a retirement village for the over 55's and I volunteer in their village Gym; it enables me to support members with their health and wellbeing both for residents and the local community. That is another big tick for my mission to support a healthier lifestyle. They are always on the lookout for more volunteers in various areas of their villages.

> **https://www.extracare.org.uk/**

When I worked as a Head of Services in Communities, Support & Care, we gave staff the opportunity to come up with ideas to engage with their customers. We ran several initiatives, and the entire workforce was given a day per year to volunteer and take part in one community project.

The Housing Officers decided to involve residents in a planting project that would improve a piece of waste land and transform it into a communal garden.

The benefits were that the community would have an improved neighbourhood and it gave the housing officers the opportunity to connect with those harder to reach customers that would only engage with our services when they needed to raise an issue. It was a really positive intervention.

This is just one idea that we put into action, however I am sure you could develop lots of fantastic ideas based on your business mission statement and how you service your customers and community. Time to get your thinking hats on.... Perhaps you could lead on approaching your employer with an idea of your own? Now that would be fantastic.

Who knows, it could work in your favour and get you recognised. It would be a great PR marketing opportunity with a good news story. It is all in how you sell it. Again, another win, win.

Don't forget to download your free copy of our 5 Ways to Wellbeing booklet which we suggest you work on after you have read the Mindfulness chapter.

Burnout to BOLD

My Ditty: I cycled a Monkey

I had spent the last few months preparing and training for what was going to be my biggest adventure yet. I started Cycling as my way of improving my physical health, I had gone from cycling around the block and feeling exhausted to being excited about starting what was an epic 500-mile bike tour from my home in Rubery, Worcestershire to Lands' End in Cornwall for the British Heart Foundation, by myself with everything I needed packed into my paneer and bags on my Orbea Mountain Bike.

I set myself a goal of cycling on average 50 miles per day. I was awake at 5am that first morning and I felt full of excitement and was looking forward to starting my journey. My destination for day one was to get to Tudor Campsite at Slimbridge, a place known to bird watchers as a beautiful part of Gloucester and somewhere I had been on a school trip as a kid. To reach this destination I would have to cycle over 50 miles.

Day One: I was blessed with crisp dry weather, and I just enjoyed the wonderful, lush countryside and the solace of cycling along, in the knowledge that I had made such great progress on my first bike tour alone.

When I pitched up at the site, with my small coffin tent, I got talking with another lone cyclist lady, she told me her story of how she was cycling from Land End to John O'Groats under her own steam. This was just the inspiration I needed to continue with my journey.

Day Two: I packed up for an early start and headed off towards my destination for the day, which was to reach

Burnout to BOLD

Brean Sands. It was a brilliant day of cycling, and I was energised to see the sea when I reached the Bristol Estuary.

During that full day of cycling, I would stop for a few power brakes, where I refuelled and rehydrated and I promised myself that once I reached my destination at the seaside, I would have a treat of a fish and chip supper. The weather was not great for this second leg of the journey, rain started to come down quite heavily, but fortunately I had a poncho that would cover my whole body.

I struggled to pitch my tent because the wind was howling, and the rain was persistent and yet I was feeling positive that I had achieved my day 2 goal of reaching my destination. The other bonus was that my legs felt good and more importantly my bum was okay in the saddle.

Unfortunately, I did not get to have my fish and chip supper, but I was simply happy to get a hot shower and dry off and snuggle into my sleeping bag, with the hope that the following morning, the weather would improve.

Day Three: I packed up my soggy coffin tent in overcast skies, I was pleased that I had got a break in the weather. I decided to head inland towards Cullompton via Taunton, where I stopped off for my lunch in a local Wetherspoons. After a few days of packet dry food, I was excited to be eating a delicious chicken burger meal.

My mobile had run out of charge and my power bank was also out of power. If I could find a plug socket I could recharge them, if only to get enough juice on my phone to use in an emergency.

Lucky as a backup plan I had taken a map with me.

Following a paper map while cycling is not always the easiest. While having my tasty lunch I used my phone to help me jot down some main villages to head towards. I then used road signs to get me to my milestones using the B roads and take the day's cycle as a real adventure.

This was my longest day in the saddle and on a few occasions, I thought to myself, 'if I am cycling in the right direction then I am still going to make progress'. My mindset was strong. I spent the day cycling and told myself I would continue to get the miles under my belt until I needed to rest up for the day and when I could find a site to camp in.

I looked out for signs for campsites from 5pm and then I came across a campsite called Digger land, which was next to a family theme park with the same name. That night I had a cup of soup for tea and decided to have an early night. Unfortunately, there was no way of charging my phone.

I went to sleep knowing that the next day I would have to revise my plan again and use the road signs to guide my way.

Day Four: When I woke up, I had accepted that this was going to be my second day of using my instincts and following a rudimentary plan to reach my destination, which was a campsite in Okehampton called Appledore.

Overall, I was having a marvellous time and I was immensely proud of myself, at how resilient I had been over the previous couple of days, and I knew that today was going to be a better day because the sun was shining.

I meandered through the countryside cycling along and

just enjoying the huge sense of freedom of breathing in the wonderful scenery and enjoying the experience. I was doing great and although my original plan and route had altered, I was still achieving my daily mileage goals.

When I arrived at the campsite, the owners kindly gave me a cup of milk, so I was able to make a real cup of tea without powdered milk and enjoy it while sitting outside my tent in the evening sun.

Day Five: My phone was fully charged which made planning my day's route a lot easier. I cycled through the beautiful Devon town of Tavistock which was immensely picturesque, and I conquered lots of hills and enjoyed the silence of the Bodmin moors and on to Liskeard.

This day's cycling was monumental on the trip because I reached Cornwall. I squealed with delight when I cycled past the road sign that said, 'Welcome to Cornwall'.

I had clocked up over 250 miles, which was half of my total trip target.

Day Six: Today was my favourite leg of my bike tour and I set off from Liskeard and hugged the south Cornwall coastline travelling through wonderful Cornish villages like Par, Charlestown, Mevigessey and on to St Mawes where I got a Ferry across to Falmouth.

It was a glorious day of weather and when I arrived at the stunning harbour of Falmouth, I decided to celebrate and stop off in the Quay to have a meal in a restaurant.

I was then faced with finding a place to camp for the night and after having such a scrumptious meal, I just wanted to find somewhere local. I did a quick google and it showed an address that was just on the edge of Falmouth. I cycled up and down the road to try and find the site with little success, so I decided to knock on the door of the address that was shown.

It was someone's house, and I was greeted at the door by a kind gentleman who explained his land was previously a site although it was no longer a registered campsite. I went on to explain my situation and he graciously offered me the opportunity to camp in his garden with the use of his toilet in his entrance hall. I was extremely grateful and accepted his offer to pitch up.

Day Seven: I moved on to my favourite Cornish Town, Hayle. It was fantastic to cycle into town to be greeted by the incredible sand dunes of Hayle Beach. I cycled into St Ives Bay holiday park with a view to pitch up my Coffin Tent in the rain but when they explained that they had Holiday chalets available I decided to book up for the next few days and use this as my base.

This was to be a great way to achieve my 500 miles and cycle around Cornwall and reach Lands' End. The beauty of this was that I was able to enjoy the comfort of a hot shower and self-catering facilities and a proper bed. I jumped at the opportunity.

Day eight, nine and ten: My husband Drew came to join me and gave me the moral boost to complete my 500-mile adventure. Having this as a base, we continued to cycle locally over the next few days, cycling to Penzance along the NCN 3 and then taking the coastal path, which was fun because it resulted in us having to carry our bikes for the most part.

The spent the next day on the golden beach and hiring a sea kayak. Day ten was about preparing to continue the bike tour and completing the mileage.

Burnout to BOLD

Day Eleven: After parking up our car, we set off in the sunshine for a full day of cycling. We visited some incredible Cornish villages on the east coast roads through St Ives on to Zennor, St Just and then Sennen Cove before reaching Lands' End.

I was delighted that I had achieved my goal of cycling from Worcestershire to Lands' End but recognised I still had a gigantic number of miles to clock up before I could fully celebrate.

As we headed inland the weather changed and the skies opened to torrential rain. We were soaked through and needed to find a place to stay. We tried a few hotels and B & B's in Marazion with little success before we found a room at the lovely Mount View hotel. We were totally grateful to be able to remove our dripping clothes and jump into a hot shower.

Day Twelve: We decided that we would return to St Ives Holiday Park and book up again and stay in one of their Chalets and enjoy the last few days of the adventure.

We then cycled the west coast of Cornwall and yes, I had exceeded my 500-mile target and cycled a monkey. I rewarded myself with a Philp's Cornish Pasty and a Cream Tea. I finished my adventure on a high, so happy to have met some fantastic people along the way.

You can find out more about our cycling adventures by visiting our Blog at:

https://jenkinsjourneys.tumblr.com/

Burnout to BOLD

Burnout to BOLD

CHAPTER 3:
CONFIDENCE & SELF-ESTEEM

This is a quality and strength that needs to be in balance. Alignment between confidence & over confidence. You can look at our bitesize animation video on my YouTube channel that explains it better if you're a more visual learner. There are several self-help animation videos to explore:

> https://www.youtube.com/channel/UCZr9P
> EY30avgHClqnw3d0Ig

Ultimately, confidence comes from knowing yourself, your worth and your abilities. Before I had poor mental health, I would have said that I was a confident person and in many respects I was. However now when I reflect, had I got the balance right?

I think it would depend on who you would ask. To some people, they would say yes and then to others they would say no. I appreciate that as a person you can always improve on your interpersonal skills and hey my whole journey has been about personal development and personal discovery in the hope that I can get better as a person.

I also recognise that if you beat yourself up worrying about this, it can negatively affect your confidence. You also must accept you cannot please all the people all the time and you should **embrace your uniqueness**.

I accept I am a people pleaser by nature, always striving to help others and yet now I ask myself can I change my approach and still help people but by doing it in a different way and being more empowering, asking more questions and taking a coaching approach to the support I offer.

Sometimes we can over stretch ourselves or as I like to call it, spreading ourselves too thin, and this could be because we are low in self-esteem and self-worth and the need to please others.

Do you prioritise your own self-worth and practise self-care above all other things, or do you cause yourself stress by over promising on your commitments in fear that people will think less of you, or have worries and concerns that you're not doing enough?

There is only you in this equation, so it is a great place to start to **get to know yourself better**. What are your strengths, are you assertive enough, whatever your areas for improvement are, how can you overcome them and stretch outside your comfort zone while still maintaining positive mental health?

It's fantastic when you get it right, it is interesting though when you look back on historic leaders or at people that are in the public eye, that there can always be a divided opinion. I am yet to hear someone that has completely got this right. So **be kind to yourself and cut yourself some slack**.

Confidence & Over Confidence

> 'Confidence' can be described as a belief in oneself and one's ability to succeed'.
>
> 'Overconfidence' can be that you have a strong bias and belief in one's own ability to the detriment of others.

Let us take a closer look at this in more detail.

Confidence is:

The state of being sure of your own ability; if you are good at something and have confidence in your own ability then this is great, embrace it. There is a lot to be said for being quietly confident. Who likes a show-off?

Feel self-assured in your abilities and celebrate them. If you are good at something, then sharing your knowledge is a great way of helping others. How does the saying go? **'Knowledge is power'**. I would say it is in how you express yourself. Think body language, tone of voice and of course your intentions behind sharing.

Have faith and trust in yourself and others: As you have already learned about me, I lost complete faith and trust in people, including my family and friends and it was an uphill climb to get this back, but if you want to succeed in anything in life, you need to surround yourself with a great team.

You must also think about your own behaviour too. For you to build a relationship with anyone you need to have the right skills for people to gain faith and trust in you too. It is a two-way street. Think about how you would like to be treated and ask yourself if you mirror that behaviour?

Have nothing to prove: Everyone has their own skill set, and some people are better at some things than others and that is great, that is the richness of life. How else can we learn and grow as people? You have nothing to prove, you can embrace being you and enjoy having the knowledge that you have. Like I said earlier, being quietly confident is a great skill, if the intentions are right.

People are often attracted to and gravitate towards charismatic people: This is an interesting word; charisma or being charismatic ultimately means that you have a personality whereby people are naturally attracted to you, you have a magnetism or quality that delights or fascinates others. Are you born with it? Or is this something that you can learn and develop?

Well, I think you can always improve how you build relationships with others; this is something we will explore further when we look at Emotional Intelligence later in the book.

Happy and joyous consistently: Are you an optimist or a pessimist, do you see joy and positivity in all things regardless of the situation or circumstance? Again, we will look at this in more detail, in 'Self-Management' in the Emotional Intelligence chapter. The key word here is consistency.

If you are on a constant rollercoaster of your mood swinging from one extreme to the other, you can be responsible for self-sabotage. Being happy and joyous will largely come from your own ability to self-regulate and ultimately on the kind of mindset you have or choose to have.

It is possible to be happy and joyous consistently and acceptance is another word that can help you achieve it.

Accept what you can change and accept what you cannot.

Sometimes things are what they are, and no amount of emotional sabotage can change it, so why cause yourself upset and worry over things that are out of your control? You will feel so much better when you encounter these things if you regulate this more. Remember, you can only change how *you* behave and hey, if others behaviour is not great that is up to them.

Radiate confidence: I believe that this is a mix of how you look, how you present yourself (including body posture), how you dress, your facial expressions and of course what you say. It is funny though, that we automatically form judgements of people within the first few seconds of meeting them, without them opening their mouths.

Perhaps we need to change our thought processes here and be more open minded and be slower to form judgements and of course be kinder. Have we walked in their shoes, do we know what their journey has been, or could we learn something from this person?

When I say radiate confidence, I mean show up, be prepared, listen, ask the right questions, and seek to understand rather than to be understood.

This is a line from probably the most well-known Leadership books of all time. The '**7 Habits of Highly Effective People'**, by Stephen Covey. It shows that this line has stuck with me because as I wrote this book, it was one of the most thought-provoking lines that I think has had a profound impact on my own self.

As I have mentioned the book, it is probably a great time to add it to your reading list. The number of people who suggested I read this book showed me that it was worth investing my valuable time into learning more. Suffice to say, it is probably one of the most respected books on personal development and leadership in the world.

Understated: This is an interesting one, because I see this as being a negative language, but it can be a positive. When I first decided to go into business, I learnt lots about branding, sales, marketing and USP's (your **U**nique **S**elling **P**oint).

In other words, what makes you or your business stand out from the crowd? After much soul searching and following a recommendation to see an image consultant, I quickly understood what it meant.

I always blended in, I chose to wear dark clothes, in fact my favourite outfit always included wearing black and dark colours. However, after learning about colour psychology, it soon became apparent that the colours that you wear can have an impact on how people interpret you, or form judgements about you.

I asked myself if the dark clothes I wore really expressed my personality. In hindsight, I would say they gave off completely the wrong impression. I then realised the importance of your image.

You can still be understated in brighter colours and exude confidence. Ask yourself the same question now, does your image express who you are, or do you need to reinvent yourself? Let us take a minute here to explore this further. Think of a time when you got dressed up in your best clothes and felt great about yourself, why was this? How you dress and show up, will impact your confidence, it is as simple as that.

So why wait to wear your favourite outfit? If it makes you feel great, then how about wearing more of the same or completely changing your wardrobe. I am not saying that you must go out and spend hundreds of pounds on a completely new wardrobe, but perhaps invest in seeing an image consultant and just getting a few statement pieces instead.

Charity shops are a great place to start. You can find

some fantastic items there, now more than ever before as people are simplifying their lives and having a clear out. We have the lockdowns and COVID to thank for that.

Assertive and balanced: You can be assertive without being overbearing, it is about getting the balance right. Sometimes in life, to protect your own mental health, we have to say the word NO.

I appreciate that this may seem negative, and I always try to focus on the power of positivity but, it is perhaps better if I say it is in how you say NO, without saying those two letters. Something like, I have commitments at this time, however I am open to discussing this further in the future and then naming a time and place or could we explore this further, I need to understand what commitment & time is needed?

The other way you can be assertive is to remain calm in situations where you feel that your opinions differ. This can result in you giving a reaction which can affect your relationship with others. It is okay to have different ideas to others, but it is about being respectful of their views and giving them an opportunity to air their opinions. We explore this further in the Emotional Intelligence chapter.

Expressive and open: Having an open mind can lead to all kinds of new & exciting opportunities. If you are confident in yourself, you can be expressive and give your opinion without being overbearing and welcome other people's opinions.

Try not to dominate and perhaps let others lead and listen to their ideas and thoughts first. You may be pleasantly surprised to hear that they have the same ideas as you. Give yourself time to listen, think and then you could form a more rounded response to any given situation.

Mindset is something we will look at in the managing change chapter. Whether you are open minded or closed minded. It could be that you will need to change your approach based on individual situations & circumstances.

The next time you are being asked to try something new, how about trying an open-minded approach, it is great for your personal development and perhaps it could work in your favour.

Authentic and true to your own values and beliefs: For me this is the most important aspect that can help you with your confidence. If you are constantly trying to fit with how others believe you should look, behave, or respond, it can be exhausting and create unnecessary stress. It is far better to **celebrate your uniqueness** and people will respect you for it.

Let us accept all our little quirks and preferences. Say you like to dress in a certain way and feel more comfortable and confident for it, then great go for it.

We all have biases, what does this mean? Well, our values and belief systems are made up from basically when we are born, they are formed generally by things we are influenced by, be it family, friends, peer groups, experiences, media (and by this, I mean, by what we have been exposed to either on the TV, on our smartphones or our environment).

Our values and beliefs are what help us develop our views of the world, the standards we live by and how we make choices. This links into how you shape your mindset. For example, if you have been brought up to have low aspirations and expectations in your abilities, the chances are you will live a life that is not fulfilling because I believe that if you have a positive mindset and are open minded to new possibilities and an eagerness to try new things, you are more likely to achieve greatness.

It is amazing that once you give yourself permission to be that fantastic person, you can achieve anything your heart desires. It's true, well it certainly is for me.

While your values and beliefs are important it is also crucial to remember that they should not hold you back from success. Just think of the most ground-breaking things humans have achieved in your lifetime. Do you think they got there from luck, or do you think it took many iterations of trying new things and pushing through and being resilient?

I can tell you now the most rewarding way to achieve success is via a journey that has helped you grow as a person and pushed you out of your comfort zone.

Overconfidence is:

Loud and noisy: Do you have to get your opinion heard; do you dominate a situation? This is what I mean by loud and noisy, it is about loving the sound of your own voice, above all else. There is a time and place for being loud and noisy and it is all about getting the context right. Who you are with and how you want to portray yourself?

If for example you are with close friends, that you know and who know you, then the likelihood is that there is trust there so you can feel confident to be loud and noisy. It is like I said, it is based on the given situation. It is good to have an awareness of this though, otherwise you might be viewed as being bullish or overbearing. Not great qualities, if you are hoping to improve your relationships and status.

Must have their opinion heard: There is a time and place for having your opinions heard and you could ask yourself, this very question next time you are in a situation when you know that you must reach new collaborative decisions. 'How can I empower others and support them with their ideas?'

It could be that their idea could bring along better results. Your opinion is not necessarily the best, although you may think it is (it may be) but give others the opportunity to try out their ideas and hey if it is not the best, you have always got that original idea you had anyway to explore at another time.

Not respectful of others' views: It is time for a bit of honesty here and you may have to do some real soul searching. Ask yourself if you are truly respectful of others' views? It is easy to jump in with both feet and talk over others when they are giving their opinion, but how about just giving them the respect, they deserve and letting them air their views first.

Okay so you may feel that your opinion is the right one and in your heart of hearts you know based on fact that it is correct but how about just taking a step back and letting others view their opinions first.

We all like to be treated with respect and think about how it makes you feel when someone jumps in and down talks your views, ideas, and opinions. It is not a great feeling, right?

You could ask yourself what would happen in a particular circumstance if you gave the other person the lead? I would suggest not a great deal, okay let us put this into perspective, I am talking about scenarios when you are with family, friends, and work colleagues. These are not life or death situations, right?

You will still have an opportunity to air your views but look at your patience as being an opportunity for you to make your case. You may have a strong gut feeling but is your opinion a rounded one? Having those few minutes and moments in a conversation can give you the time you need to formulate your response.

Remember, it is also okay to say, I need time to consider and reflect on your views and I will come back to you. So perhaps what you could do is clarify what the timescales are to move the project or scenario on. If you are strong in your holding of your view, this will then give you the breathing space that you need to get further information, be it facts and figures, consultation with others or even support from others that share your view.

Sounds like a good idea, I would say. Does this help? Respect is key for building great relationships and productive communication. Overconfident people that rush in, without giving that respect, are evidence of how lack of respect can be damaging.

Unsatisfied and unhappy: Are you a natural pessimist, do you get frustrated and have a low mood consistently in all things regardless of the situation? Overconfident people may be unsatisfied or predominately unhappy with other aspects of their lives.

This links specifically into your mindset, which we will cover later in the book. How you moderate your moods and thoughts will help you build your confidence, whereas overconfident people may get hot under the collar and can blow their tops at the smallest of things.

This is a great opportunity to again do some soul searching, I now say to myself if I am in a certain situation whereby, I feel that I am getting frustrated or even angry. 'Hey, it is what it is. You can have your opinion and I can have mine'. It is okay that we can agree to disagree.

Happiness comes ultimately from being self-assured and confident in your own abilities, so do not let unhappiness creep in and consume you. Find joy in the small things.

I once read the book '**Eat that Frog**', by Brian Tracy which is about procrastination and getting the important things done first. I took a lot out of this book regarding unhappiness and happiness. It helps to put things into perspective.

Have low self-esteem: Firstly, it helps if you understand what self-esteem is so that you can look at it more subjectively.

Self-esteem is about an individual's subjective evaluation of their own worth and about how your belief system influences your behaviour. Looking at your levels of empathy for others for example. If you have low self-esteem, which might be an underlying issue in some overconfident people, then it is unlikely to make you an extremely popular person.

Have you heard of **Maslow's Hierarchy of Needs** (Maslow, A)? Let me explore and explain this in more detail.

In real people's terms the Maslow's hierarchy of needs is a motivational theory in psychology. It comprises a five-tier model of human needs, often depicted as hierarchical levels within a pyramid. Needs lower down in the hierarchy must be satisfied before individuals can attend to needs higher up this will affect your levels of self-esteem.

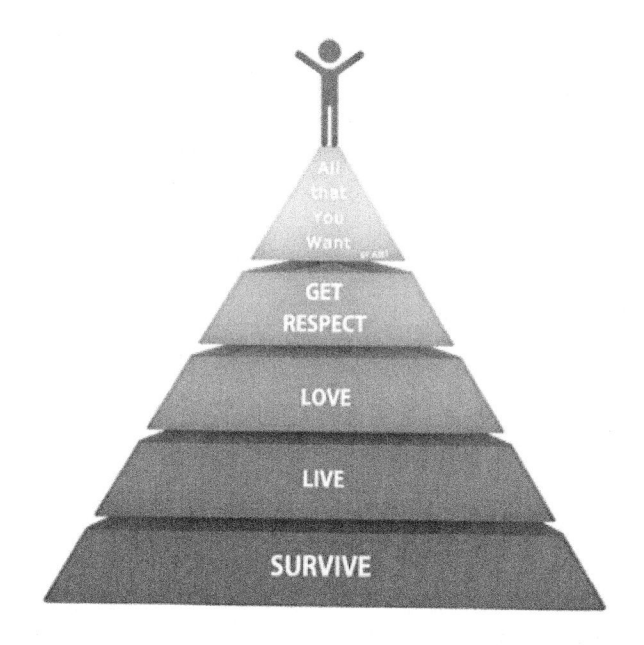

Pyramid diagram with levels from bottom to top: SURVIVE, LIVE, LOVE, GET RESPECT, All that You Want, with a figure standing on top

Often not factual and tend to make stories up:
People that are overconfident may make things up on the fly to better themselves and big up their own abilities. It is far greater to be prepared and have knowledge of the facts once you have done the research as this will help you to increase your confidence.

Having a story is important especially in the landscape of entrepreneurship for example. Rather than making it up, it should be prepared and practised to support you in giving your message. For me, my story is based on the premise of this book, my journey to improve my own Mental Health and Wellbeing. This could be a good point for you to find your story or stories?

What does this mean, well, you may not have had an experience like me that has been a pivotal point in your life, but you may have had points in your life where you have had to overcome adversity or times and experiences that have shaped who you are.

It is okay if you are not entirely confident in knowing what your story is but take a look at my YouTube channel or listen to our Podcast, where you will find an interview with local Businessman Ernie Boxall from Ernie Said that might make things clearer for you.

https://www.youtube.com/watch?v=uI3L9rCRWkY

Ernie is a specialist in helping people develop their stories, using the 4 P's method of perfect presentations. Ernie believes you should **'Turn up, Stand up and Speak up'**. Speaking is a skill you can learn and the more you develop your story, the more confident you will become.

Criticise others: Overconfident people may criticise others without being subjective and putting themselves in the other person's shoes. It is a good idea to check in with yourself before criticising others.

Everyone has their own journey and who they are will be different to you and your journey. If we could all be a little kinder and less judgemental then maybe, we could get along better.

Confidence is about having confidence in yourself and your own abilities. You will find that people are trying to be the best versions of themselves as a rule and if we could be more tolerant and subjective then it will help you build your confidence.

Sensitive and can have verbal outbursts: Do you take time to check in with yourself? Do you understand your hot triggers? This is a good place to start for increased confidence, do you pause before you speak? Or do you feel that you must jump in and have verbal outbursts?

It is far better that you are measured when you are responding to others and remember that what they say is not personal, so being more objective is the right way to react. This is all about emotional intelligence and something we will explore further on in this book.

To put this into perspective for you, I will give you an example of my journey.

When I was experiencing poor mental health, I would often have verbal outbursts and be particularly sensitive. Blaming others for my situation rather than taking responsibility for my current state.

There was one memory when I had disagreements with my family and rather than being objective, I became overly sensitive. This resulted in disagreements and more full-blown arguments.

This is not helpful to anyone. This just made my self-esteem and confidence tumble more. Is this something you could relate to?

Take a more confident approach when you find yourself in a situation where things could escalate and take a moment to practise mindfulness.

Full of self-doubt: Are you constantly doubting yourself and your abilities, are you more pessimistic or optimistic? Over-confident people may be more likely to play down their strengths for fear of being outed as an imposter.

Imposter syndrome is a psychological pattern in which an individual doubts their skills, talents or accomplishments and has a persistent internalised fear of being exposed as a "fraud".

This manifests itself in the need for perfectionism. Perfectionists set excessively high goals for themselves, and when they fail to reach a goal, they experience major self-doubt and worry about measuring up.

Success is rarely satisfying because they believe they could have done even better. That is neither productive nor healthy.

This is a good point to ask yourself these questions:

- ♥ Do you micro-manage people?
- ♥ Do you struggle to delegate tasks and responsibilities?
- ♥ Are you allowing your self-talk to play down your achievements?
- ♥ Do you often experience burn out and feel that you must work harder?

Now you have asked yourself these questions try turning them around to:

- ♥ How could I empower people more?
- ♥ Could it be far better for my Wellbeing if I delegated more?
- ♥ If I focus more on my successes and the positives, then I could be more confident?

- ♥ Do I need to practise more selfcare to enable me to achieve my goals?

This will increase your confidence by looking at the positives and having the right mindset.

Must be the centre of attention: Have you ever walked into a room and found that there is someone in there, that is dominating and loud? Over-confident people often like to be the centre of attention and have a big ego.

Attention seeking behaviour is said to demonstrate someone with a personality disorder, it comes from a need for admiration and validation.

That said, there is a time and a place for you to assert your dominance for example when you are giving a talk or speech, but it is far better to be reflective and mindful. This approach is much better for personal development.

Heightened Self Esteem: It is useful at this point for me to define what self-esteem is; self-esteem is used to describe a person's overall sense of self-worth or personal value. In other words, how much you appreciate and like yourself.

Self-esteem can play a significant role in your motivation and success throughout your life. Low self-esteem may hold you back from succeeding at school or work because you do not believe yourself to be capable of success.

This again is an issue that requires establishing a healthy balance. When you have healthy self-esteem, it means you have a balanced, accurate view of yourself. For instance, you have a good opinion of your abilities but recognise your flaws.

Comfort Zone

Overconfident people often stick within their comfort zones, where it's easy to stick with the status quo. However, for good personal growth and for you to achieve your full potential it is worth moving from your comfort zone into your stretch zone from time to time.

There will be circumstances when you need to stick with your comfort zone, and this is for you to decide from a wellbeing perspective. There are some things to consider like your response to certain situations when it can affect your stress and anxiety levels.

Reaching your goals, hopes and dreams often requires you to move outside your comfort zone and learn new skills. Move into your stretch zones and growth zones.

Ultimately, the reality is that once you have stepped out of your comfort zone, you will have developed as a person, this is a continual journey, one that can help you achieve greatness in whatever you want to do in life. We all have that inner voice that talks to us.

My favourite book that looks at this is **'The Chimp Paradox'**, by Prof Steve Peters. In it, the author helped me to recognise that I was the person that was holding me back and how I had been letting my emotions dictate my life.

We all have inner voices and I found that the loudest voice was the negative one. By listening to both a positive chimp and a negative chimp, you can balance this out and choose how you want to respond and let the positive voice win.

It is only once I recognised the chimps' voices that I was and still do, take it as an opportunity to reflect and give myself time to think things through.

Reflection

Having time for reflection is necessary for us to grow. Reflecting helps you to develop your skills and review their effectiveness. It is about questioning, in a positive way, what you do and why you do it and then deciding whether there is a better, or more efficient, way of doing it in the future.

By writing down the thoughts that we keep in our head, we can gain clarity that helps to create our vision. Getting your thoughts on paper can help you understand why you are feeling a certain way and make those feelings a little easier to navigate. This is a balancing act because while reflection is a positive thing to practise, it is important that we move on.

To effectively use reflection, you need to be honest with yourself and objectively observe yourself as a third person. We can all identify times when things have not gone as we would have hoped, and that is okay, if we learn from it and improve it for the future.

We should also use reflection when things have gone well, this helps us to celebrate success and understand why things have gone well, so you can replicate it more in the future.

Celebrating successes is important to our wellbeing because it releases our happy hormones in our brain and helps to create a positive mindset so we should practise celebrating more.

Visit our website for our FREE downloadable 'Reflection Handout':

Our website is
www.advanceyourwellbeing.co.uk

Burnout to BOLD

My Ditty: Egg on my face

I took a deep breath and stroked my lap to straighten my red dress, as I sat there waiting for my name to be called. I had spent the last month rehearsing my talk, repeatedly and yet as I sat there my mind was in complete turmoil.

I reached for my mobile phone to try and help me regain composure. I read and reread the notes on my phone, then suddenly, I woke as if coming out of a deep sleep. "Welcome to the stage, Marie Jenkins".

Oh, my goodness, it was my turn to give my talk. I stood up to a welcoming applause and walked towards the stage. My heart was racing, and my hands felt clammy. I turned to face the audience and was greeted by a sea of smiles. So why was it that I felt so completely consumed by nerves?

I had given several talks to large crowds of people, on many occasions previously and some were in difficult circumstances with a hostile crowd, when I was a Head of Service.

I felt completely inadequate and incompetent in a room full of people who were there to do the same as me, which was to hone the craft of becoming a professional speaker.

I began my introduction with a smile and the whole time I had this internal dialogue going on. I tried to catch my breath and focus on what I had been rehearsing repeatedly. I knew exactly what I was going to be talking about because I had lived my recovery from poor mental health, so why had my mind gone completely blank.

I opened my mouth, and nothing came out. I stood there and tried to gain composure and started to mutter and stutter words and I am not exactly sure how much sense these words made.

I continued with the talk and as I looked out to the people in the audience and locked eyes with one of my fellow speakers the worse thing happened.

I completely froze. My mind went blank. I stood there like a rabbit caught in headlights. I kept opening my mouth and nothing came out. My heart was in my mouth, and my emotions were out of control.

I then uttered the words, 'I'm sorry, I cannot continue with the talk', I vaguely remember different people in the audience shouting out, 'It's okay, just gain your composure and you will be fine'. I knew this was not the case. 'I'm sorry, I'm just not ready for this'.

I then found myself walking back to my seat, what happened next was a blur, people were talking to me with words of encouragement and support, but I just felt like I was in an out of body experience.

I could not hear any of the positivity, all I could focus on was the complete sense of being a failure. I felt like I was going to vomit with nerves and yet I just continued to sit there and smiled and apologised for wasting everyone's time.

Looking back, I now know that it was too soon on my journey back to recovery and my confidence and mindset were not yet ready or that was the narrative I had given myself at that time.

Did I really have egg on my face or was it just my

negative view of myself and my abilities?

I have since learnt to be kinder to myself and accept things for what they are. It really is incredible that the narrative we give ourselves determines our successes.

Burnout to Bold

CHAPTER 4: MINDFULNESS

What is mindfulness?

When I was on my road to recovery from poor mental health, I learned about mindfulness. Well firstly I learnt to give myself time to calm my over thinking mind. I was in a constant state of awareness, over analysing everything. I felt I had lost my purpose. So how did I switch my mindset?

Instead of having a victim mindset and seeing things negatively, I decided to switch things around and take responsibility and ownership of my life and have a more positive mindset.

Once you do this, you will find your relationships will improve and people will gravitate towards you. **Positivity breeds positivity** and it is true.

Think about when you were in a room filled with people, who were the ones you found most drawn to, was it the person that was all doom and gloom or was it the person that had a can-do attitude, radiates positivity and is happy in nature? I bet it was the positive one, right?

Since switching my own mindset, my life has transformed. I have also learnt to accept things outside my control, like other moods, and concentrate on the things in my life I do have control over. Such as my thoughts and feelings, my future direction.

When I did this, things began to happen for the better. Your mood can affect an atmosphere, so it is a good idea to check in with yourself and choose the right mindset for your day.

I then put mindfulness at the centre of my life, living in the present moment, being grateful for the important things in life such as my health, my relationships and having a roof above my head.

Life can accelerate us forward at a pace that means we

are in automatic pilot or going through the motions rather than doing things with purpose and focus. It is far better to take things slowly, giving yourself time to reflect and reassess your priorities. This is the real essence of living life mindfully.

> **Our mind can have up to 6,200 thoughts per day, (Tseng, J., Poppenk, J. 2020) and recent studies have shown that this number can increase when your body and mind are under stress. A large volume of these thoughts can have a negative effect on our actions. It is important to concentrate on the more positive thoughts and that is where mindfulness can help you live with purpose.**

How you react and overreact

Mindfulness is about living in the present moment and without judgement. Quite often we rely on others to bring us happiness and if we are feeling stressed or anxious, we can react to situations or circumstances without a balanced view.

This can lead to catastrophising and adding to our stress levels and from here it can be a downward spiral of negative thoughts and over reactions.

If we are feeling tired or exhausted, we often over think and begin to distort our thoughts and feelings and lose all sense of reality. Mindfulness can help you in these given situations to check back into your emotions and tune in to how we are feeling.

Our emotions inform how we react or overreact, and we will look at this in more detail in our Emotional Intelligence Chapter. By practising mindfulness, we can give ourselves the opportunity to be more subjective and prevent the doing mode or living in autopilot.

Regular meditation or periods of mindfulness has many health benefits, it can improve your memory, cognitive ability and it can aid your physical & mental health.

> **Research has shown people who practise mindfulness on a regular basis are more likely to be healthier, happier and more content and less irritable with more improved relationships, you can find more information about this research by visiting University of Oxford Mindfulness Centre website.**
>
> https://www.psych.ox.ac.uk/research/mindfulness

When I was struggling with my mental health, I accepted the use of medication from my doctor and while I appreciate that for some medication is a lifeline, for me I just felt even worse, tired, and sluggish and I felt I was sinking even lower into my depression, and I was losing perspective as to what reality was.

Then I discovered mindfulness, in fact it was an audible book by Mark Williams and Danny Penman; **'Mindfulness; The eight-week meditation program for a Frantic World'**, *that completely turned things around for me.*

I took the holistic approach to recovery from then on after weaning myself off the medication (something that you should always take advice on) and for me it really worked. I am now a massive advocate of mindfulness and continue to practise it every day in many different forms, which I will go into in the practical ways later in this chapter.

Accepting difference and tolerance

We can all be guilty of having prejudices or preconceived notions of others, research shows we often judge people, solely on their appearance, basically within the first seven seconds of meeting someone new *(Association of psychological science. 2011.)*.

This can lead us to conclude their trustworthiness, whether they are honest, all sorts of things like their values and beliefs. This can then inform our levels of tolerance towards them and whether we would like to form a relationship with them.

It may be far better to practise mindfulness and be more accepting of their differences and turn our mindset around to help us grow and be more open minded because the reality is we can learn something new from every encounter we have and from every conversation.

Taking a more open minded and positive mindset, we can check back in with ourselves and frame things in a different way. Like, by asking ourselves, **'What could I learn from this person and what could they teach me?'**.

Differences can bring us together and it is the richness of difference that can bring about positive change, innovation, and fresh ways of thinking, including creativity.

We can all be guilty of being judgemental, it is what makes us human. It could be far better for your own personal development to be more mindful.

Typical scenario is, you are at work, and you have been invited to join a new team and while you may know you already like most of the team it's just that one person, you're unlikely to get along with. You have already formed a judgement that you are unlikely to get along with them if you must work together.

This approach is nonconstructive. How about reserving your opinion and investing in time to get to know the person on a deeper level, removing the emotional aspect out of the relationship can be far better for your own mental health.

In life there will be people that we do not necessarily like or want to spend time with, that's life, however in a work environment this is different, we may not always be able to choose who we do or do not work with. You will still have a responsibility to work together cohesively and collaboratively.

> **Visit the NHS website to find out more about practical ways to use Mindfulness**
>
> https://www.nhs.uk/mental-health/self-help/tips-and-support/mindfulness/

Practical ways to use mindfulness techniques

Before I share with you my practical mindfulness techniques, I thought I would share with you some benefits of practising mindfulness on a regular basis.

1. Beneficial to your mental and physical health
2. Calm the overthinking brain.
3. Gives you time for reflection.
4. Time and space for new thinking.
5. Awareness of your surroundings and getting back to nature.
6. Thankful for your loved ones and what you have.
7. Living in the present moment.

1. Benefit to your mental and physical health:

When I was in school, I was always keen on PE, I was part of the netball team, I took part in trampolining, cross-country running and loved to swim, somehow between then and 2013 I had fallen out of love with my own selfcare and in fact myself.

I was on a treadmill of life putting everyone else's needs before my own. Can you relate to this? Historically, the connection between physical and mental health has been largely unexplored and now it is evident that both are interconnected and impact on each other.

> **The Mental Health Foundation has a great pdf that you can explore further:**
>
> https://www.mentalhealth.org.uk/publications/how-to-using-exercise

Fundamentally the essence of the link between the positive impacts on your mental health through physical activity is about the sense of feeling good and our ability to thrive with all life's ups and downs.

Your emotional state is still likely to be impacted by life's natural experiences such as grief, loss or failure and success. However, being physically active can help you lead a more balanced and mentally healthier life.

You only have to turn the TV on now and you are bombarded with weight loss adverts or slimming and dieting plans and of course we all know about Joe Wicks, the nation's PT teacher.

> https://www.youtube.com/c/TheBodyCoachTV/videos

We have become a nation obsessed with the need to be slim, is this the way to demonstrate great health? We assume that slim people are healthier, and it could well be that they are internally healthier than those people who are overweight.

With Wellbeing, this goes a lot deeper. If you are looking to achieve wellbeing, you have to look within. I am going to ask you to take a few moments to ask yourself what you believe Wellbeing to mean? Grab a pen and my handout 'What wellbeing means to me', yes seriously I want you to do this now.

> **Visit our website for our FREE downloadable 'What wellbeing means to me':**
>
> **Our website is**
> **www.advanceyourwellbeing.co.uk**

This is important to do because wellbeing means different things to different people.

Now read back to yourself what you wrote. If you have put anything material on your list, then cross it off and start again in the second box. Then give yourself time to come up with ideas on how you can get there.

It may be that you put your initial thoughts down and revisit it once you have given yourself some headspace. That is okay, although it is important that you do complete this because it will help you when you look at the 5 Ways to Wellbeing Booklet (that we mentioned in the earlier chapters).

2. Calm the overthinking brain:

How many of us take our smart phones to bed and check in to our social media channels before we try to go to sleep? I would say a high majority of people.

I was one of those people. It would be the last thing I did at night and the first thing I would do in the morning. Especially when I was at the height of my mental health crisis.

I was over analysing all my friends' interactions; I had become consumed with who was saying what and who was interacting with who? I had become completely paranoid.

Looking back now, I would say that I was experiencing paranoid schizophrenia, although this was not clinically diagnosed. I do not want to fill you with fear. It is important that if you are reading this and have concerns about your mental health it is important to get professional help. There is a lot of help out there and I would suggest you get in touch with your GP in the first instance.

On reflection this was not helpful to my wellbeing, and I now recognise that you cannot control other people's behaviour, you can only control how you react to it.

If you are in this position and you can relate to this over-thinking brain, you need to STOP and check in with yourself. That is where mindfulness comes in.

Like I was saying at the beginning of this section if you are taking your smartphone to bed now is the time to complete a health check. How do you do this?

> **Visit our website for our FREE downloadable 'Health Check Handout':**
>
> **Our website is www.advanceyourwellbeing.co.uk.**

Most of us need 8 hours of good quality sleep to function properly. It is important to have a healthy bedtime routine. When I was experiencing poor mental health, I would often have periods in the night when I would wake up with lots of thoughts rushing through my mind.

I then took a notepad and pen to bed and if I woke up with my mind racing, I would jot my thoughts down. This then allowed me to switch off and go back to sleep.

Poor sleep habits can be a risk to your health and wellbeing. Good sleep gives your body and mind the opportunity to recuperate, repair and boost your immune system. Here are my top tips to improve your sleep.

- Tech-Free bedroom: Leaving your phones out of the bedroom and have your bedroom as a place for rest and relaxation.

- Light and temperature: Have the right mood lighting that creates a relaxing environment, low watt bulbs or bedside lights. The temperature of your bedroom can affect your ability to sleep well, be aware of what your preference is.

- Stressing over a good night's sleep: The more you will yourself to sleep, the more likely you are to have a heightened sense of awareness. If you are struggling to sleep, get up and go into another room, make a cup of tea or a milky drink and sit peacefully or meditate. Then when you are ready, return and try again.

- Food & Drink: Try to avoid having caffeine-based drinks, as this will make you more alert and try to have meals more than 3 hours before you plan to go to bed, this will give your digestive system the opportunity to process any food you have eaten, this will help you fall asleep faster.

- Alcohol consumption: Alcohol can make you feel tired, however as the effects wear off, it can impact on the quality of your sleep. Finding that you are more likely to wake needing to visit the toilet or rehydrate your body with a drink of water.

- Exercise Regularly: If you have regular exercise, it is more likely that you will have a better night's sleep, also avoid exercising late at night, as your body is likely to have a boost to its adrenaline production and this can hinder your ability to relax and ultimately fall asleep.

- Avoid Napping: If during your day, you take a nap, then this will affect your ability to have a full night's sleep. If you are feeling fatigued during the day, take yourself out into the fresh air, go for a walk or do something that could stimulate your mind, like a puzzle or play on a computer game.

- ♥ Sleep Diary: By keeping a diary about your bedtime route and the quality of sleep you had, it can help you to identify the best conditions and routines that aid a great night's sleep.
- ♥ Calm your over-thinking mind: Try and relax while lying on your bed, avoid the temptation to let your mind race about any worries or anxieties you have, instead let it wander and try to drift into memories of happier times or things you are looking forward to.

3. Give you time for reflection:

Do you race through life, chasing your tail feeling that your life is on autopilot? It is useful to give yourself time to reflect, then you are investing in your own personal development, you can evaluate what you have achieved, what has gone well, what you could do differently and improve for next time.

Reflection can help you process your thoughts and feelings and give you the breathing space you need to overcome any challenging situations, that said it can also help ground you, if you have had success.

I have developed a handout that you can use on a regular basis, for example perhaps on a Sunday evening before you start a fresh new week, or on a Friday when you have had a full week of work. It may be that you do this handout monthly, whatever works for you.

> **Visit our website for our FREE downloadable 'Reflection Handout':**
> **Our website is**
> www.advanceyourwellbeing.co.uk

Then after doing this exercise on several occasions, you will be able to identify what your tendencies are, what you need to stop doing and what you could do with building on or has worked well.

Many cognitive behaviour therapies include reflection in mindfulness because it helps individuals to connect with their emotions and regulate them. This can help you prevent catastrophising, which is where you view a situation as being a lot worse than it is. This can have negative effects on your mental health.

You can then switch your mindset, to explore how you could do things differently for a more positive outcome both emotionally and physically. The mindset you choose to have will deliver results; we will explore mindset further in our Managing Change Chapter.

4. Time and space for new thinking:

By practising mindfulness throughout the day, it can give you the time and space you need to develop new thinking and improve your wellbeing. I can hear your cogs whirring from here. What has this got to do with Wellbeing?

> *Okay stick with me here, let me take you to Christmas morning when you were a little kid.*
>
> *You woke with a huge amount of excitement to see what Santa had put under your Christmas Tree, you leap out of bed, filled with curiosity and hopefulness, and launch yourself down the stairs to see a fabulous array of beautifully wrapped gifts.*
>
> *You had no idea what you were about to find, however you were still filled with sheer delight and wonderment of what you were going to discover. You unwrap your presents and lay them to the side. You then find yourself playing with the boxes more than the gifts themselves. This is where your creativity kicks in.*

It seems to me that as adults we are so focused on achieving the end goal and that we have forgotten the art of play and the benefits that this has on our wellbeing.

That is why it is so important to give ourselves the time and space we need to do this more often. There are lots of research papers out there that show that children have less fear and more imagination than adults and this is partly because as adults we do not access our divergent thinking like we did as a young kid.

This is because as we have grown, we feel we need to conform to norms to fit into society and this can have a massive impact on our wellbeing. The more we give ourselves time to try new things and permission to experiment the more confident we become.

> **Watch this TEDx Talk on YouTube from Elizabeth McClure**
>
> https://www.youtube.com/watch?v=g00o6LCmaMI

With increase in confidence, you may well make better decisions and life choices. Look at the book '**The child's right to play: A global approach'**, by Rhonda L Clements and Leah Fiorentino.

5. Awareness of your surroundings and getting back to nature:

I have always been a lover of the great outdoors, I would say most of my life's holidays have been spent camping, be it near a seaside location or in a countryside setting, and this got me wondering as to why I would naturally choose this as my preferred holiday?

After carrying out vast amounts of research it has been no surprise to me that by submerging yourself in nature it can improve your wellbeing, both physically and mentally.

We take our beautiful countryside quite often for granted yet when we take ourselves out into nature, we automatically feel more relaxed and calmer.

The fantastic thing about nature is that we can find it and nurture it wherever we are. Be it from a walk, run or cycle in our local parks, or from growing plants and vegetables in our gardens or houseplants indoors.

Have you ever heard of the word 'Ecotherapy'?

Ecotherapy is an approach that rests on the idea that people have a deep connection to their environment and to the earth itself. By practising ecotherapy more it can massively improve your mood, your inner emotions and promote your sense of wellness.

I cycle every Sunday and naturally choose routes that enable me to submerge myself in nature. This is my opportunity to practise mindfulness, I take in huge gulps of air, and it feels like a big dose of nature's medicine.

I always feel so much better. I clear my mind and leave my worries behind and live in the moment. It really is the best way to improve your wellbeing and there are always new things to discover, learn about and experience. Get yourself off the settee and try it and experiment with doing it in a mindful way.

> **Visit MIND website to find out more about ecotherapy:**
>
> www.mind.org.uk/information-support/tips-for-everyday-living/nature-and-mental-health/about-ecotherapy-programmes/

6. Thankful for your loved ones and what you have:

Recently I watched the movie Cast Away with Tom Hanks, and it is a fantastic film that demonstrates human resilience, determination and the sheer will to survive.

The premise of the film is about a man who was

marooned on a desolate island for four years, with no means to escape. While it was not based on a true story, there have been a few stories in history that have been similar. It always gets me thinking about how I would have survived and thrived in a similar environment, especially as you are completely on your own with no-one to share it with?

As humans we are sociable creatures, with **a basic need to belong**. The need to belong refers to the idea that humans have a fundamental motivation to be accepted into relationships with others and to be a part of social groups.

The fact that belongingness is a basic need means that human beings must establish and maintain a minimum quantity of enduring relationships. We need this interaction to help us feel connected, accepted, and supported.

Loneliness is a hot topic now, and I can imagine everyone has been affected by this at some point during the pandemic. Your mental health is massively affected by your feelings of being part of a group, community, or sense of belonging.

I can put testament to this because when I had poor mental health, I cut off from everyone, my friends, and my family. This is not great, not by any stretch of the imagination. It took my journey to recovery to help me to recognise this.

I now make it one of my main priorities to ensure I am **staying connected to the people in my life** and I am hugely grateful for them. These are two of the elements of the **5 Ways to Wellbeing** that I spoke about earlier on in this book; 'Connect' and 'Take Notice'.

I now have a great network of people in my life, with varying degrees of knowledge and skills that I can call on and hopefully support them too. It is important to nurture your relationships and the film Cast Away is a great reminder to me that we must be thankful for all the people we have around us.

Mindfulness practice helps to shift unconscious behaviours that impact your relationships. Since many of your behaviours and responses in relationships are conditioned and habitual, shifting them in positive ways takes more than conscious effort.

Mindfulness practice helps to make these shifts. It is about being accepting of others' ideas, opinions whilst removing your biased views.

Ask yourself, how you are as a friend or family member. Are you reliable and trustworthy, are you open to others' ideas? Next time you are having a conversation with someone, press pause on your need to respond and share your opinion and just take time to listen in its truest sense.

You never know when you might need to call on that person for help, it is always good to be more thoughtful and kinder.

Many people have heard and read the book, '***Men are from Mars and Women are from Venus'***, by John Gray. This is an excellent book because it helps us to understand the different psychological differences between the sexes. We could all do with learning more about this so that we can cultivate successful relationships.

The other book I would recommend reading is David Ricoh's book, '***How to be an adult in relationships; The five keys to Mindful loving'***. He says, "Most people think of love as a feeling, but love is not so much a feeling as a way of being present." It certainly makes you question and have a fresh look at how you love and find relationships.

7. Living in the present moment:

How many of us are constantly thinking ahead, be it new goals or things that you want to achieve? These are all vital elements that as humans we need to have, things to work towards and strive to accomplish.

The thing is, with us constantly looking ahead we sometimes forget to live in the present moment, and really take notice of all the things we have in the here and now. This is how mindfulness can help us calm our over thinking mind.

If we are constantly thinking ahead, it can cause anxieties and worries about the big mountains we need to climb, and it can feel too enormous and that is why we can get side-tracked or put things off all together.

Many people say it is about the journey not just the result and whilst this is true, we must find a balance. Celebrate all the wins that we achieve along the way as well as the big mountain climbs, that will massively help you.

My question to you now is, **'What are you thankful for in the here and now?'** Do you take time to really look at your life and reflect on all the wonderful things you have, be it relationships, health, and your own sense of being?

Well, there is no time like the present to do just that. I have created a **'My Gratitude Notes'** handout for you to capture your thoughts and feelings and the things that you're grateful for?

> **Visit our website for our FREE downloadable 'Gratitude Notes Handout':**
>
> **Our website is**
> www.advanceyourwellbeing.co.uk

Being grateful can be massively beneficial to your mental wellbeing and there are several ways you can practise gratitude. Here are a few ideas.

Observing, how many times during a day, do you say the words 'Thank you'? Is this a habitual response or do you mean the words you say? Think about when someone shows you gratitude, it gives you a warm glow inside, you feel valued and appreciated.

Take notice of the things you are saying thank you for, the act of kindness that is shown, and try to replicate this in your behaviour. It can be massively rewarding and improve your wellbeing. As well as improving your optimism it can give you great pleasure.

Share with others when you have received acts of kindness, it is infectious and can help others feel valued.

Tune in to your senses: the ability to touch, see, smell, taste, and hear, how often do we take these abilities for granted? How many of us have our moods lifted when we receive a hug or a stroke on the arm from someone we love. It is immensely powerful, the sense of touch.

Many of our emotions are impacted by what we see, this is one of the senses that has a gigantic impact on our wellbeing. The wonderful sights and scenery we get to enjoy in life is all through our eye's lens.

Think about when you have been aroused by a gorgeous smell, be it the smell of fresh bread or a lovely home cooked meal, a perfume or cologne or the bouquet of a fine wine or fresh bunch of flowers.

Taste, now we all have a particular food or meal we enjoy, remember when you had a cold as a kid, and you lost the sense of taste. It totally affects your appetite. In our diverse culture we get to have our taste buds boosted with flavour. How fantastic is that?

Our hearing is a massive sense when it comes to our ability to communicate well with others and our enjoyment of music, film, and comedy. By tuning in to your senses, it can help you to recognise how valuable our senses are to us and the joy it brings to your life.

Pets: There has been an increase in people getting new pets during the pandemic and it is massively beneficial on so many levels to have something other than yourself to take care of, as well as them being a fantastic companion.

I am not advocating that you should rush out and get a new pet, because it is a huge commitment, however if you have given it plenty of thought then it can bring so many rewards.

Physically, by improving your health by going out on walks (dogs) and mentally because they can reduce feelings of loneliness and enable you to get in touch with your emotions.

Having someone to hug and love and bring friendship. This might sound odd to some but for me my dog Bourbon is like my best friend, he gets to hear all my ideas before anyone else, he is an excellent listener, and he is always happy to see me.

Pets come in different shapes and sizes, and for some small pets like fish or budgies can bring equal happiness to larger pets. Whatever works for you is the important thing.

Have visual reminders: Create a visual storyboard of all the things in life that make you feel grateful and happy. It could be people, places, or special items like a sentimental item that you received from a loved one.

Every time you look at your visual storyboard, it will make you smile and release those happy hormones.

> *Without getting into too much science here, your happy hormones are what your body creates and that flow through your blood steam. They play an important role because they help to regulate your mood and produce endorphins, which are your body's natural pain reliever, and your endorphin levels tend to rise when you engage in reward producing activities. (Take control of your health with no-nonsense news on lifestyle, gut microbes and genetics. 2021).*

Make a pledge; This is a pledge to yourself, one where you pledge to practise self-care and show gratitude to others. I have something that can help you make these pledges.

> **Visit our website for our FREE downloadable 'Pledge Card':**
>
> **Our website is**
>
> www.advanceyourwellbeing.co.uk

The best book I have read, that helped me with my over-thinking mind was **'Mindfulness'**, by Prof Mark Williams & Prof Danny Penman. It is an eight-week programme, and it can bring calm to your mind.

It may seem a bit airy fairy to some, and I was possibly one of those people that believed that meditation was something that hippy types do, however if you go in with an open mind you will find it does work, whatever role you play in society.

Remember mental health is something that every human has, and it can affect anyone, regardless of your background, affluence, and status.

Let me refresh your mind, that we are looking at things differently now without judgement and with greater acceptance and tolerance. The hippy type of comment is a fine example of bias and a brushing statement. It is easy to make comments and statements like this and this just shows how easy it is to do.

Burnout to BOLD

My Ditty: The horse has bolted

My knuckles were white as I clung on to the reins, my leg was waving around while my foot looked for the stirrup. I had lost my navy and white boater shoe and I was clinging on for life as the horse bolted. I was petrified.

The day had started off so differently, I was so excited because the farmer had offered me the opportunity to exercise his beautiful black stallion on his land.

I was on a family caravan trip in Cornwall with my brother, Mom, Dad and Nan. Along with Bonnie and Clyde our liver and white springer spaniels. We had been on the site for a few days and today was the first day that we had wonderful sunshine. It was ideal weather to go on a pony trek across the lush green fields of his farm and around his fishery that was on the other side of his land.

"Have you ridden a horse before?" asked the farmer's wife. "Yes", I replied. I was 13 years old, and anything seemed possible to me at that age. I had never had official riding lessons, yet I had exercised a friend's horse on several occasions; basically, I had been on the horse for 3 weekends for an hour each time.

What with that and the traditional organised pony trekking excursion when we had been to Butlins on holiday and the donkey rides on Weston beach as a youngster. I felt totally confident, climbing into the saddle, and taking a stroll around the farm on his beautiful animal.

The farmer's wife introduced me to Pippin, their black stallion. It towered way above me and yet this did not phase me. "Come with me, climb on out here", she guided me to some steps in the yard and I climbed on board.

My brother and Dad were looking on, as they had been

making their way to the fishing pond with their rods in their hands for a morning of fishing. Once the horse tack was altered to make for a comfortable ride, she led me to the gate and guided me as to where to go.

Pippin and I then trekked across a long grass track that had been made previously on the field. At that moment, I can honestly say, I was a happy 13-year-old, living in the moment, enjoying the excitement of being in charge of this huge beast.

Many people would like to practise mindfulness in this kind of situation, although at this age, I was just being a carefree teenager.

I found myself talking to the stallion as we plodded along, and I was clicking to usher it on, as it kept stopping to munch on the long grass. We reached the bottom of the field, and I pulled on the reins to guide the horse towards the other side of the field and then within a blink of an eye, the horse bolted. Galloping at full pelt.

By the time, we arrived at the gate by the yard. I was in complete shock. Pippin had decided that once he turned, he could see the yard and knew that was where his food was. How on earth had I managed to cling to the stallion and survive without a broken limb?

I climbed off the horse and found that I was breathing heavily. My legs had turned to jelly, and yet I felt exhilarated. I was okay, still intact.

This was just one of my childhood memories that I remember with fondness. When I returned to the caravan, I found my mom, Nan and the dogs sat there, and I retold my experience and they just laughed. I then joined them in a rupture of laughter.

This was just another life affirming stories that shaped my life. I am sure you have them too. What are yours?

Burnout to BOLD

Burnout to Bold

CHAPTER 5: RESILIENCE

What is resilience anyway?

The definition of resilience is *'**The capacity to recover quickly from difficulties, toughness**'*.

I always thought I was a resilient person; I could face most things and find positives, then everything changed when I had a period of poor mental health. It led me to question everything in my life; my relationships, my purpose, my why, my reason for being. Was I even resilient in the first place?

I had lost all the resilience I had, or thought I had, and everything was stripped away. You may be at this pivotal point yourself.

Now this is where I am going to show you some tough love. Let me tell you here and now, if you feel like you're not resilient, let me tell you, you are and you can absolutely build this back and become stronger as a result. They say **what doesn't kill you makes you stronger** and as someone has been through a huge amount of personal development in recent years, I can tell you, this is so right.

The reality is I was resilient; however, I had never been in this circumstance before and so I felt I had gone back to zero, however I found the courage to recover so I must have had a degree of resilience.

Your vulnerabilities are your strength, and your life is a journey with hopefully few lows and many highs. It is the rich tapestry of life. When you have had everything stripped away this is an opportunity for you to build yourself back as a better person for your own sense of self and to be a better person for others.

Showing compassion, generosity, and empathy to others, while nurturing your own wellbeing and finding your inner peace. I know I am in danger of sounding all peace and love here. I know Utopia does not exist and terrible things go on in the world. The pandemic and atrocities teach us this.

When our mental health suffers, we can get into a state of catastrophising. If we try to take all of life's burdens on our own shoulders it can be a slippery slope. Something we should navigate from.

The point is you can only be in charge of your own thoughts and feelings, you need to concentrate on the things that are within your control, that is not to say that you can't have passions and hold your own strong views and opinions it's just to say, find your own inner peace, and happiness will return to your life.

It is important to note that I am not a psychotherapist, I am sharing with you my insights based on my own personal journey and what has helped me.

There are some great books on Resilience. I would recommend you read '**The Resilience Club'**, by Angela Armstrong; you can also find it on audible. I enjoyed listening to this while I was driving between business meetings.

What I would say is, that it is filled with lots of useful tips, and you might do what I did and find yourself pulling over to capture the ideas. Sometimes it's worth doing both.

Having a paperback and listening online. It's whatever suits you and your way of learning. Angela has some great resources that accompany her book via her website, that cover topics like how to maintain high performance, and high energy, and help with decision making.

You can access Angela Armstrong's website here:

https://www.angelaarmstrong.com/book-

Childhood

Your childhood experiences will have shaped your resilience in the here and now. To give this some context, I said earlier that I felt I was resilient, I grew up looking back with a high level of empowerment, I had freedom to choose what I did, pretty much. I hear people call it things like feral. Left to be wild. I choose to put it in its positive context of being empowered.

Now that said I have not always felt that way, yet now when I look back, I am glad I had the childhood I did because the resilience I had built up has helped me to overcome what was my darkest time. It is important to note that your own personal resilience is like a changing spectrum.

Your levels of resilience will alter depending on many different factors like the situation, your ability to build relationships and the circumstances you're in. Your childhood experiences will also have a bearing on your current levels of resilience.

Sometimes the toughest life experiences can be positive because they can help you to be more resilient in the future.

You only have to watch the news today to hear the huge number of concerns for our younger generation and how the pandemic has been detrimental to their mental health and how school closures may result in years of missing out on their education.

Let's move away from this negative narrative and find the positives. You could argue that this generation will come out of this pandemic much more resilient and will have learnt new skills that will support them to thrive in life's lows and highs. Especially in their future careers because the world of work is changing, and they would have certainly learnt about the skill of independence.

What is more important for children for the future? To be more rounded, adaptable to change and understand the importance of self-care? Or to carry on as we have been doing whereby wellbeing and our mental health has been second to our thirst for academic know-how?

Academic knowledge is hugely important, but it is also about getting the balance in life. Now hopefully we are moving more towards this for us to gain the knowledge we need to achieve our dreams and aspirations.

Okay so this doesn't help you now, I get it but take time to think about your childhood. The things that you experienced and how it has shaped you as a person. I have developed a '**Childhood: My Personal Experiences'** handout that I think is now a great time to use and reflect on.

> **Visit our website for our FREE downloadable 'My Childhood Experiences Handout':**
>
> **Our website is**
> **www.advanceyourwellbeing.co.uk**

You could also read Rick Hanson's book, '**Resilient: Find your inner strength**'. He shares his experiences of his childhood and how it helped him to shape his compassion and his adult life. Rick poses that anyone can build up resilience, the key to a positive mindset, an unshakeable sense of self and the ability to get back up again and withstand anything life throws your way. He has distilled 40 years of clinical work and teaching into 12 practical, highly effective tools to help you build your resilience.

Values and beliefs

Our personal values shape our experience of the world. So, I'll ask you this question; **Are your values and beliefs holding you back from moving forward?**

Acceptance is one thing that can help us move forward with a better mindset. When I say acceptance, I mean looking at self-acceptance and acceptance that others will have different sets of values and beliefs to you and find the positives in this and embrace them.

> **Conscious awareness of our values can stop our brain from producing overwhelming amounts of cortisol: the hormone which, when produced under pressure, stops us being able to think clearly it can cause the brain to shrink (A, Mitchel. 2016). This then can result in us feeling anxious and stressed. You can see that holding strong values and beliefs can be detrimental to your Wellbeing.**

Freeing your mind of your strongly held beliefs can help you be alert, think freely and be more patient and find more fulfilment and joy in life. Let's explore your held values in more detail. I have created a '**Values and Beliefs to Positive Behaviours'** handout to help you move to more positive behaviours and be more productive and happier.

> **Visit our website for our FREE downloadable 'Values and Beliefs to Positive Behaviour Handout':**
>
> **Our website is www.advanceyourwellbeing.co.uk**

5 Pillars of Resilience

The **'5 Pillars of Resilience'**, (G, Mathias.2021) is a great model to help you build yours.

Many areas of the 5 pillars have already been explored within other chapters in this book.

1. Self-Awareness
2. Purpose
3. Selfcare
4. Relationships
5. Mindfulness

1. Self-Awareness

To be more resilient it is useful to be more self-aware. In terms of how you are feeling in any given situation or how you respond to others.

Your thoughts and feelings are always within your power to control. The best way to learn more is to write a diary, looking at your strengths and areas for improvement.

Trying new things is a great way to explore this further, how you coped and reacted to any given situation.

2. Purpose

It is important to have a purpose. For me it was about starting my businesses to help people achieve their full potential, for you it could be completely different; like being better in your job or improving your health and wellbeing.

That's why it is a great idea to set yourself new goals and aspirations. Start by jotting down 5 new things you want to achieve this year in the space below. Then focus on them, what do you need to make them a success?

1.

_____

_____

_____

2.

_____

_____

_____

3.

_____

_____

_____

4.

_____

_____

_____

5.

_____

_____

_____

By breaking larger goals down into smaller manageable bitesize chunks you're more likely to be able to achieve them.

C. Selfcare

It is important to practise self-care on a regular basis, it is what will help you become more resilient, reduce stress and be more rejuvenated. If you have higher energy levels, you will be more focused and happier.

Selfcare can be taking time out of your day, to do something you enjoy, it can be eating a healthier diet, or it could be just taking your dog out for a walk. Whatever it is, find your happy place and invest more time in doing that.

D. Relationships

Resilience empowers and sustains healthy relationships, having good social relationships is clearly a winning strategy in life, tied to greater psychological and physical well-being.

Thus, it's not surprising that social relationships also matter when it comes to resiliency, in part because they help us feel less stress when we are suffering.

Invest time in the relationships you have and prioritise building better relationships.

E. Mindfulness

I then put mindfulness at the centre of my life, living in the present moment, being grateful for the important things in life such as my health, my relationships and having a roof above my head. Resilience can be built when practicing mindfulness and it goes hand in hand with self-care and self-awareness.

Life can accelerate us forward at a pace that means we are in automatic pilot or going through the motions rather than doing things with purpose and focus.

It is far better to take things slowly, giving yourself time to reflect and reassess your priorities. This is the real essence of living life mindfully. You will become more resilient because of it.

Positivity & Facing your Fears

Are you a positive person? Are you an optimist or a pessimistic person? Or as the saying goes, a glass half empty or a glass half full kind of person.

Your outlook on life will help navigate you to greater things. If your outlook is more, 'woe is me', then you may tend to attract the most negative things in life, it's basically a downward spiral.

You can be absolutely in control of your future success by simply switching your mindset. Think positive, be positive and talk positive. The language you use is often a reflection of how you're feeling, so take time to check in with yourself.

People tend to gravitate towards those people that have a can-do attitude and see the brighter side of things, this is purely because positivity is something that people find attractive in a person, and they like to emulate and learn from you.

Comfort Zone, how often do we live in our comfort zones, that place where we feel safe and at ease?

I would say overall we do, it's our human default setting and our way of feeling confident and is an easy road. You are not alone in living that way. However, the last year of the pandemic has taught us **we are more resilient and capable of far more than we ever imagined** if we face our fears and move from our comfort zones into our stretch zones.

From a personal growth perspective, it is useful to step outside of our comfort zones and practise stepping into our stretch zones more and that includes when the pandemic is over. This is where you will realise your full potential and go on to succeed in something that could pleasantly surprise you.

There is a balance to be had here, in terms of stretching more, whilst recognising that you do not stretch too far and end up in your panic zone.

This is where you over stretch yourself and end up with negative impacts on your wellbeing. Staying in the stretch zone is where your personal growth will develop, and it is where most of the learning will take place. So how does it feel to be in your stretch zone?

It may be scary to begin with, and this can transpire in physical reactions like butterflies in your stomach or feelings of nervousness and that is completely normal. This is when you need to check in with yourself and give yourself permission to give new things a try. Remember failure is not true failure it's an opportunity to learn, understand more about yourself and build on your strengths and most importantly build on the area's you're not as strong in.

Many people will have experienced the Dunning-Kruger Effect, whereby people overestimate their abilities.

> **You can watch a short video on the Dunning-Kruger Effect by David Dunning.**
>
> https://www.ted.com/talks/david_dunning_why_incompetent_people_think_they_re_amazing/transcript?language=en

The reverse of this is the imposter syndrome, this syndrome refers to an internal experience of believing that you are not as competent as others perceive you to be. This is where self-awareness is key.

People with the Impostor Syndrome are highly critical of themselves. This often results in a strong pressure from themselves to excel and this can often be found in people who are high performers.

Take a read of Laura Whitmore's book, **"No one can change your life except for you"**. In it she shares her experiences of overcoming heartbreak, body image worries, self-doubt, and insecurity. Laura has learned that optimism, self-belief and learning to accept yourself, will bring you more than anyone else can ever give you.

Progress over perfection should be something that we focus on achieving. How many times in your life have you come up with some fantastic ideas but that's where they start and end.

They are basically just ideas because you're spending so much time on thinking of the big goal and how wonderful and shiny it would be once you have achieved it. That you spend more time procrastinating rather than beginning. This is where progress should win over perfectionism.

It is important to have that big Dream for sure and I am a huge advocate for having those dreams, however like everything in life, great things generally do not happen overnight.

Now some people are extremely lucky in terms of hitting the ground running and creating overnight success, whereas most of us must put all our blood sweat and tears (hopefully not too much, because where is the fun in that?) into a goal or dream.

Look for the positives here, if everything was plain sailing and it came easy, would you still find the passion, interest, and drive to keep going? **The things that seem harder to achieve are often the things that help us grow as people in relation to building our resilience, growing our knowledge, and honing our skills**.

Having high standards is definitely a good quality to have if this helps you move forward, whereas perfectionism can hold you back. How about just thinking to yourself, 'let's do the best job I can at any given time, see what the feedback is and what reactions I'm getting and then fine tune and improve as I go along'? That way you are sure to make progress.

There will be bumps in the road, or as I like to say it's more of a roller coaster ride, sometimes you get the lows and then other times you get those amazing shots of adrenaline when you have achieved something incredible.

The trick here is to acknowledge those highs and lows, making sure they don't consume you or change who you are as a person unless it is for the better.

This is where you can sink to having bouts of feeling

useless or poor self-esteem as you go through the lows, or you can have an inflated ego when you're riding through the highs. ***It is important to remain balanced and humble.***

My Ditty: Blood in the Swimming Bath

Gasping for air, I surfaced from what was an aqua swimming pool, to what looked like a sea of red. I was dazed, my legs were peddling with ferocity, and I gulped air.

Earlier that day, I was looking forward to our PE lesson because we were going to be learning lifesaving skills in our swimming lesson. I always enjoyed swimming as a young kid, and every Saturday we would visit various leisure centres with my brother, nan, and grandad.

My nan was never a great swimmer and I remember she would try and do a breaststroke and sink deeper with every stroke, which would leave my brother and I in fits of giggles.

My grandad on the other hand was always a strong swimmer and would encourage me and my brother to feel confident in the water and become strong swimmers. By the time I was a teenager, I was able to swim for lengths and lengths of a pool.

'Come on girls', we heard Mrs Richards shout through to us, as we got ready in the changing rooms. The buzz in the changing room was one of fun and excitement. I was always very sporty at school and was an active member in numerous different teams and clubs.

The girls I was with that day were also like me, and we were looking forward to this swimming lesson. We stretched into our speedo swimsuits, grabbed our goggles, and dashed out to the pool side.

The first part of the lesson went well, you know the type of lesson, when you had to pick up a rubber brick from the deep end and swim through hoops and see how far you could go under water holding your breath. We were called by Mrs Richards, to sit at the side of the pool and she explained that we were now going to do swimming circuits of the pool to measure our distance ability.

We sat there dripping wet, waiting patiently for our turn to be called. We then lined up and you were invited to either jump in or dive into the pool and follow the swimmer in front of you.

Michelle stood in front of me, and as we dithered waiting to be directed into the pool we chatted about usual things, like our arrangements to go shopping at the Kingfisher centre that Saturday or what we thought about the music charts on Sunday.

Duran Duran was my favourite band and hers' was Wham, we would often compare our Smash Hit magazine and exchange our icon's images so we could cover our schoolbooks or stick up the pictures on our bedroom walls.

We were then aware that it was our turn to get into the pool, "Michelle, go.", She stepped forward and jumped in. "Marie, go.", without concentrating I moved to the side and put my feet on the edge and launched myself into the pool diving headfirst.

'Crunch'. That was my memory of the sound I heard in my head as my face entered the water and Michelle's foot made contact with my nose. Then the rest was a blur, until I surfaced from the water.

"Are you okay, Marie?", Mrs Richards, was stood above me at the side of the pool, 'swim to the steps and get out of the pool', What was going on, all I could see was the blood that had congealed around me, my face felt numb and as I wiped my face to remove the chlorine water from my eyes, I could taste the blood on my face.

As I climbed out of the pool, I was guided back to the changing rooms. I looked at myself in the mirror and was shocked to see that my face had ballooned up, my eyes were almost closed due to the swelling and blood was still dripping from my nose. I was numb to the pain because the adrenalin was still pumping through my body.

I thought to myself, my nose was broken. The teachers made the necessary arrangements, and my mom was called. As it turns out my nose had been broken and what followed was two lovely black eyes and continual nose bleeds. It resulted in me having to have my nose cauterised to try and stop the ongoing nose bleeds I was experiencing.

They say that your resilience is built up based on your childhood experiences, and this was just one story of when I needed to be resilient and move forward and learn from my mistakes.

I should have taken more notice of the teachers that day, instead of chatting with my friends in the line. I could have been more mindful of what was happening in the pool before I dived in.

While this was an event that left me with a lump on my nose. It certainly helped to build my resilience. I learnt that sometimes things happen, and it was an opportunity to build my strength of character.

I am sure that you have also experienced things in your life that have helped you build your resilience, and it could be a great chance for you to reflect on how you overcame them and what your coping mechanisms are.

Burnout to Bold

CHAPTER 6: EMOTIONAL INTELLIGENCE

I was lying on a sun lounger in Cyprus when I first discovered the concept of Emotional Intelligence.

Someone I knew had recommended that I read **'Emotional Intelligence 2.0'**, by Jean Greaves & Travis Bradberry, and it put a lot of things into perspective for me. It was like a light bulb moment, in terms of what Emotional Intelligence is and how I could learn more to improve my relationships and ultimately be a better person myself with others and most importantly for myself.

How many times in your life have you had those pivotal life affirming times? Well, this was one of those times for me. It was after listening to this book on audible that I recognised that I had spent my whole life as a people pleaser, putting others before myself, both in my career and in my personal life.

How was this helpful to my own mental health? In fact, I would go so far to say that this new learning was a real game changer for me and my life going forward.

In this chapter I am going to be exploring Emotional Intelligence, in more detail in the hope it has as big an impact on your life for the better as it did for me.

EQ and Science

I will try my best not to get too academic in this section, although I do believe it is important to understand more about how our brain works and how it can affect our physical actions and behaviours.

One of the best thought leaders in this field, among many, is Daniel Goleman and he has written many papers on EQ (Emotional Intelligence) and Social Intelligence.

He has a PhD in Clinical psychology. His book **'Emotional Intelligence: Why it can matter more than IQ'**, is a fascinating read. With new insights into the brain architecture underlying emotion and rationality, Goleman shows precisely how emotional intelligence can be nurtured and strengthened in all of us.

Emotional intelligence is the ability to understand, use, and manage your own emotions in positive ways to relieve stress, communicate effectively, empathize with others, overcome challenges, and defuse conflict. The great thing about EQ, is that you can improve it as you learn more. Here's the science part.

Emotions are not just a matter of the heart. Recent advances in research have shown that they are also a result of brain biochemistry. These conclusions come from neuroscience, evolution, medicine, psychology, and management. Most scientists believe that the control centre of emotions in the brain is the limbic system. The limbic system stores every experience we have from the first moments of life.

Brain circuitries tell us that the brain is affected by our emotions in two ways:

1. *Signals travel from the first brain to the rational brain and then back to the emotional brain whenever we mull something over for a while and become increasingly angry, determined, or hurt. The "mulling over" allows us to receive more precise data, and this leads to good decision making and more effective actions.*

2. *The second pathway is the route the signal takes as it travels to the emotional brain before going to the rational brain. This occurs when there is an immediate and powerful recognition of a specific experience as the emotional brain makes an association with some past event; we react strongly to something without really knowing*

why.

The brain seems to have one memory system for ordinary facts and another for emotionally charged events. Emotional events appear to open additional neural pathways that make them stronger in our minds, which may explain why we never forget significant events.

Occasionally we are propelled into action based on these few rough signals before we get confirmation from the thinking brain. We have a rational brain that keeps us from being overpowered by strong emotional reactions, but the emotional brain should not be completely overshadowed by the rational one. The key is balance.

(Emily A. Sterrett, 2014)

Self-Awareness

Our ability to learn more about emotional intelligence can be split into different areas. Having higher levels of self-awareness, can help us regulate our emotions and more importantly manage our behaviours.

When we can recognise our moods, or emotional states, our drivers for our behaviours and our triggers then it can help us to monitor and identify our levels of self-confidence, help us to assess our emotional state and have higher levels of self-happiness.

Let me give this some context. If you're reading this and feeling that you don't feel fulfilled in your current life or career choice, then now is the time to start looking at yourself and making some pretty life changing decisions.

Are your values and motivations aligning with your current path?

Need I say more? Well, here are some other ways being self-aware can help you:

- ♥ It can help you to recognise your core strengths, the things you really excel in and the areas that you're not so great at. Then you can learn more and/or do things differently.

- ♥ When you have a heightened level of self-awareness you are more likely to feel motivated to act.

- ♥ You can recognise others' perceptions and moderate your behaviour; these are qualities you find in great leaders for example

- ♥ You can build better personal & work relationships, by having a greater emotional awareness of how your emotions affect your behaviour, reactions, and responses in any situation

- ♥ It can help you to question yourself and find your true passions, the things that get you out of bed in the morning, the things that give you the determination and motivation to see things through. If you are passionate about something, you more likely going to have additional resources in your wellbeing bank to see you through those less successful times.

- ♥ It can help you concentrate on things you take enjoyment from and perhaps delegate to other things you enjoy less.

I appreciate this is not always possible and you will have some tasks you enjoy less than others but once you have a heightened level of self-awareness it will give you the resilience you need to complete a less favourable task.

I for one am not a big fan of washing up, so I got a dishwasher. And when I spoke to a coach about this, he said he enjoyed doing the washing up because he used it as his time to practise mindfulness.

Sometimes we all have to do things we wouldn't necessarily choose to do, but they have to be done. It's worth doing those less favourable tasks first, say at the start of the day and then moving on to the more favourable one's after.

This is guaranteed to boost your happy hormones, one because you have achieved the one thing you don't enjoy and secondly because you were able to spend more time on doing the things you do.

Having high levels of self-awareness gives you the tools of self-control. It can be extremely empowering, in terms of your own abilities (internal self-awareness) and how you build effective relationships (external self-awareness). This is what we will focus on more later in this chapter.

The first step to self-awareness is about understanding how self-aware you are, that way you can find your starting point and build on it.

When I was recovering from poor mental health, I took multiple self-awareness tests. I guess I was my own best task master. I was looking for the 'Holy Grail', the one thing I could change to be this better and more well-rounded person.

These tests come in different forms. Some people call them personality tests, others use psychometric tests and others use Leadership assessments. I guess which one you choose will depend on where you're at in relation to your health, career, and personal life.

Self-Management Strategies

One of the best self-management strategies is to prioritise your own health.

Being physically fit is as important to your mind as it is to your physic and your muscles. A healthy way of life will positively impact your mental health.

Self-Management strategy 1

Keeping yourself hydrated by drinking plenty of water may seem like an obvious thing to do, how many of us keep a track of our daily intake?

Following research, recommendations say that women are advised to drink 2.7 litres of fluid and men to drink 3.7 litres of fluid per day (Healthline. 2021. **How Much Water Should You Drink Per Day?**).

An easier way to keep a track of this is to think of 8 cups per day. Being well hydrated helps to improve your sleep quality, helps to keep your joints lubricated, increases cognition and your mood.

From an emotional intelligence perspective if you're physically well, you're more likely to be able to focus and improve your relationships.

Self-Management Strategy 2

Keeping journals or diaries, this is an opportunity to put down all your emotions and feelings about any given situation (L, Billingham 2021).

You can be honest with yourself by doing this, without burdening your close family and friends. Many of us now use digital means to record events and post about our preferences and observations but there is something more mindful about writing down our thoughts and feelings.

You could start by using your journal to capture how you feel about the day. Did you feel that overall, your wellbeing was in a great place, or did you have experiences that you felt could have been better?

By writing this down you can track each of your more positive emotions and build on the things that you feel have hijacked your positivity. The other benefit of keeping a journal is that you can capture any ideas that you get throughout the day and then follow them up with action.

Self-Management Strategy 3

Be interested, how often do we have a conversation with someone with our whole purpose about giving a response. Instead, perhaps it could benefit your emotional intelligence to *just listen* and put pausing and breathing techniques in before your response?

People like to feel valued and that their opinion matters. You can do this in a variety of ways, count to 3 in your head before your reply or ask more questions, another idea could be to put yourself in their shoes.

By trying to see things through someone else's lens, it can help to build trust, empathy and help to connect. This is an easy strategy to practise every day.

Self-Management Strategy 4

Vocalising your goals can be a great way of holding yourself accountable. When you put things out there, into the Universe, it can be a great start to your journey. As humans we can have hundreds of ideas, ambitions or goals that just stay exactly that. By vocalising them, you have a sense of responsibility to work towards them.

There are different ways of vocalising your goals, it could be to share with a family member, a work colleague or with a mentor and some people can choose to share them to the world and that is okay too.

It's up to you to decide what is right for you.

Self-Management Strategy 5

Be prepared for success. When you have goals and dreams, you can be so focused on achieving that end goal that when you reach it, and you achieve success it can result in a heightened sense of emotion.

Having a healthy ego is important, although it is useful for you to check in with yourself and manage your emotions. You want the success to be a positive experience for all involved.

Take a look at the Success Cycle model. This is when you set your goals, check in with your feelings and emotions, take positive action and then analyse the results. A book that explores the success cycle model in more detail is, **'The Success Cycle: 3 Keys for Achieving Your Goals in Business and Life'**, by Marques Ogden'.

Social Awareness

Are you like an open book, do you keep all your emotions and thoughts and feelings on show?

This can be demonstrated by your facial expressions (A, Carter. 2021) and tone of voice more so than what you say, your body language and posture and your facial expressions.

It may not be that obvious to you at first, but the reality is that people will get their social cues from how you react in these various ways. If you allow yourself to be so transparent, it can influence how people react and engage with you.

This is about recognising and understanding the emotions of others and regulating your behaviour to meet the needs of others.

Social awareness is about your abilities to connect with others, recognising their emotions and adapting your behaviour accordingly.

The best way to do this is to set yourself a goal to observe more, be it from a far or when having a conversation with others. To increase your social awareness, it is important to be present, so what do I mean by this?

Think about a time when you were in the middle of a conversation when someone outside of your circle interrupted you or when the other person decided to take a call rather than ignore it and be fully present. I can imagine this made you feel less important and not valued? When I say be present, I mean be fully focused on that person, avoid any distractions.

Now I bet you're reading this and thinking it is obvious, but once you tune in to it, and start practising being present, you will be amazed at how easy it is to get distracted.

The best example of this is at home when your partner comes in from work and you ask how their day has been and the kids come running in to gain your attention. The dynamics quickly change, and what often happens is that you forget to check in with the individual on an emotional level and the conversation gets left behind.

Your five senses are there for a purpose and you can use them to build your social awareness as well as your sixth sense which in this case is your ability to recognise emotions in others. There are a few ways you can pick up on these signals or cues.

Social Awareness Strategy 1

Your whole identity is defined by your name or nickname, when people use your name or remember your name, you feel valued, it creates a sense of belonging and helps you be more connected.

It is incredible how using someone's name can positively influence their behaviour and reaction and help towards building a relationship.

Social Awareness Strategy 2

A person's eyes can tell you so much more about what a person is thinking and feeling more than any other part of the body.

Being able to have great eye contact with someone can help to connect you. It can show that you're sincere and that you care.

Social Awareness Strategy 3

Timing is everything. Observing other people's moods and deciding when best to approach them can make all the difference in the outcome.

How you frame your question could have an impact on the outcome however their frame of mind will also have a massive impact on the result.

Pick your moment; when you can or change your approach, by offering support or showing empathy, it can help to connect you and give you an opportunity to address the questions you originally had, at a different time. This is about focusing on others' moods and not on yourself.

Social Awareness Strategy 4

Catch the mood of the room. When attending a meeting or event, you can often pick up on the atmosphere, rather than multitasking by taking notes or using your phone, give yourself an opportunity to home into the other people, that are there and observe, notice their facial expressions, connect by using eye contact and simply listen more.

Remember that **social awareness is about them not you**.

If you are due to attend an event, go with an open mind and live in the moment and plan. Have some conversation questions prepared to help you to engage with new people or continue to build relationships with those people you already know.

Social Awareness Strategy 5

Drop by to say 'Hi', quite often our interaction with

others is built on a hidden agenda, following up on a previous task or conversation or asking for help or achieving an objective.

Sometimes it's the less formal conversations that can help you to build those stronger relationships. Just speaking or calling someone up to ask how they are doing with no other reason can be the most effective in terms of social awareness. People will value your time and effort and welcome an opportunity to tell you something that they have been working on.

Again, it is about them not you, so by doing this, they feel more valued and are more likely to open up to you about other things.

Relationships

Most people put the biggest amount of effort into a relationship when they first meet or as some people call it during the honeymoon phase.

The reality is all relationships take constant effort and work. For those people that make a concerted effort in building and maintaining their relationships, they are more likely to have deeper and enriching ones.

Your relationship with others should be about inspiring others, helping them to build and grow and your ability to bond closely. By being curious and selfless with others you can help to improve the relationships you have in your life. Add value where and when you can, this will help to strengthen your bond.

Try not to be judgemental of other people's choices and decisions, instead be open and curious. It is a good point to recognise your own personal style and understand how people see you here, for example if you're a positive and fun person to be around, build on this, people will naturally gravitate towards you.

Relationship Strategy 1

Avoid giving mixed signals, consistency is important to help people build those lasting relationships. Do what you say and say what you mean.

Stick by your core values and beliefs, that way people will understand who you are as a person, and it will avoid confusion. This will help to build relationships that are meaningful and help with communication.

Matching your tone and what you're saying to your internal emotions, will also help to build relationships.

Relationship Strategy 2

Remember the little things. Think of a time when someone has done something for you, no matter how small and when they gave thanks or praise. It makes you feel good inside, right! By doing this in return it can have huge benefits to your long-term relationships.

Being grateful or having gratitude can help to remind us of the simple pleasures in life. Those key moments in your life and probably the best memories you have, will be based around being with someone and sharing an experience. Take time to notice these and appreciate them for what they are.

Our lives are filled with these small moments; however, they often get lost in the busyness of life and that is why it is important to capture them and give thanks for them. I have developed a **Gratitude** handout for you to capture these special moments, we just need to train our brains to recognise them more often.

Visit our website for our FREE downloadable 'Gratitude Notes Handout:

Our website is
www.advanceyourwellbeing.co.uk

Relationship Strategy 3

Good Old-Fashioned Manners, is something that us Brits are renowned for, however in today's society how often do we use these words flippantly without giving them further thought or meaning, for example at a shop we ask for something and you say, 'Thank you' or 'Please'; do we mean it or are we just saying it?

The same goes for when we have done a great job at work for one of our colleagues, do we take it for granted or do we use it as an opportunity to pay a compliment to other colleagues and show recognition?

Spreading positive vibes creates a happier relationship so how about let's all recognise this more and cherish our manners and use them for what they are intended for.

Relationship Strategy 4

Be open to feedback. If someone comes to you with feedback positive or constructive, do you automatically have a default response? For us to build stronger relationships it is important to actively seek out feedback, rather than to wait for it to come to you.

Other people's feedback is the best source of information in terms of personal development we can get, it helps us to see how others view us and you can take this learning and either build on the positives or mitigate and or alter the not-so-great feedback.

Relationship Strategy 5

Build Trust, the bedrock of any relationship has trust at the core. It is important to remember that trust is one of the key components of any successful relationship and it can take time to build, although it can be empowering to give trust right from the start of a relationship.

During the pandemic, leaders of Organisations have had to give trust to their employees to work remotely.

With the future of how we work being a hot topic we now have an opportunity to reinvent our workplaces and place trust at the heart of everything and redesign our management principles.

There is a great book called **'Reinventing Organizations'**, by Frederic Laloux that explores the TEAL approach. TEAL (Technology Enabled Active Learning) is a theory that empowers employees to self-manage and develop a culture and help grow a business, without the need for hierarchy, based on peer relationships.

How can you build trust? To gain trust you must also be prepared to give trust. Some people believe that trust is earnt over time, here are my top tips in building trust

- Respect the privileges you have been given
- Have integrity
- Ask for help when you need it
- Take responsibility and be accountable
- Explain your thought processes to others
- Avoid gossip and emotional responses and keep to the facts.
- Be consistent
- Make rational decisions
- Show vulnerability
- Be sincere and authentic

There is something that can help you measure trustworthiness, and it is called the Trust Equation, this can be quite complex.

> You can access a great blog from Jostle on: Ways to build trust at work:
> **https://blog.jostle.me/blog/ways-to-build-trust-at-work** . It has some great practical tips and examples to help you understand how you can build trust.

My Ditty: And the winner is....

How did I get here? were the words I muttered to myself under my breath. I was dressed up in the most beautiful red dress, my hair was groomed, and I had a face full of makeup. I felt great and at the same time, I was having like an out of body experience.

Wondering how I had got here. I looked around at the most stunning venue, which was in an art deco style. The table we were sitting at, was a formal dinner table with lots of amazing business professionals seated all around me.

I was at the Midlands Business Awards at the Athena which is an incredible venue that was originally a cinema in Leicester.

My business had been shortlisted for an award in the category of Innovation of the Year. I was feeling immensely humble and appreciative to have gotten this far.

After completing an application, I was invited to sit across from a judging panel of fantastically successful Midlands Business owners that were at the top of their game. After making it through this stage, I had been shortlisted for the award and invited to this wonderful glitzy event, to hear if my new business was going to be recognised.

'The winner of the Innovation of the Year goes to', were the words I heard that made me sit up and take notice. As the host Harj Sander read out a list of other businesses in my category, I heard squeals of delight and raptors of applause going on at various tables around me.

Then it was my turn, 'Marie Jenkins from Advance your Wellbeing', everyone around me on our table cheered in support. I felt my face flush red with a mixture of embarrassment and pride. I could feel my heartbeat in my chest.

'The winner is….', well, my name was not called, and I was okay with that. I was just so amazed that I had gotten this far, especially as my Business was still in its early stages, as it had been set up just a couple of years ago. In business terms, it was still a baby and I also had lots to learn.

The reason I tell this story is because it shows how my emotional intelligence has developed. Just like it could for you.

Rather than catastrophise, I was able to look at the positives. I had not won the award; however, I had been able to learn from the process, and was given the opportunity to raise awareness of my fledgling business to a room filled with successful business owners.

There are always positives and that's where your self-management comes in.

Burnout to BOLD

Burnout to Bold

CHAPTER 7: MANAGING CHANGE

Are you reading this book because you have reached a pivotal moment in your life where change is needed in order for you to move forward? I can appreciate that change is an extremely difficult thing to overcome but it can also be empowering.

When I was recovering from poor mental health, I had to make decisions about what I needed to change in order to achieve what I wanted in my personal life and my career.

How you manage or approach personal change will have a massive impact on your wellbeing and I for one can attest to this. The mindset you have will be the difference between being able to move on positively or falling into a downward spiral, where negativity breeds negativity.

How ever you look at it, the latter option is not great. Remain focused on what's within your control.

Mindset

Your Mindset is a set of beliefs that affects how you think, feel, and behave, the key is not about ability, but your beliefs about your ability. Pro C, S, Dweck identifies two mindsets:

1. Fixed Mindset

2. Growth Mindset

You can read more in Prof CS Dweck's book, ***'Mindset, The new psychology of success'.***

Fixed Mindset

A fixed mindset could prevent you from fulfilling your potential. Your view of yourself can determine everything. If you believe that your qualities are unchangeable (the fixed mindset), you will want to prove yourself correct over and over rather than learning from your mistakes. People with a fixed mindset tend to have static intelligence, avoid challenges, give up early, believe that effort is fruitless and see feedback as negative although criticisms can help us grow. A fixed mindset can leave people threatened by others' successes.

Growth Mindset

A growth mindset can help us achieve our full potential and propel us forward to achieve success. People with a growth mindset tend to have dynamic intelligence, embrace opportunities, have persistence in face of adversity, believe that effort is a pathway to honing a skill or craft, and see feedback as an opportunity to develop and grow.

A growth mindset can help you feel inspired and celebrate other people's accomplishments and learn from others.

You can change your mindset although it does require practise and a big helping of self-awareness. The most successful people have a great insight into their own strengths and weaknesses and tend to have a growth mindset.

Look at the book: **'*Extraordinary Minds: Portraits Of 4 Exceptional Individuals'* and *'An Examination of Our Own Extraordinariness'*,** by Howard, E Gardener. In these books Gardener explores the different types of intelligence. Perseverance and Resilience are the two common competencies found in those people with a growth mindset.

Now is a great time to ask yourself what type of mindset you have? I have developed a quick and easy **Mindset Test** handout looking at intelligence, creativity, health, and wellbeing and much more.

> **Visit our website for our FREE downloadable 'Mindset Test':**
>
> **Our website is**
> www.advanceyourwellbeing.co.uk

Opportunities or Challenge

How you view the world can determine your mindset and the language you use can also represent your thoughts and feelings. Let's look at opportunities and challenges, are these the same or are they different?

My favourite quote is from Winston Churchill, he said:

A pessimist sees the difficulty in every opportunity; an optimist sees the opportunity in every difficulty"

What does this say to you?

This is just one example of how language can frame our feelings, the English Dictionary defines challenge and opportunity as:

Challenge: A challenge is something new and difficult which requires great effort and determination

Opportunity: An occasion or situation that makes it possible to do something that you want to do or have to do

You can see that the word challenge has negative connotations, whereas opportunity has positive connotations. People with a growth mindset are more likely to favour an opportunity over a challenge.

There are various theories from Linguists on language and human cognition and whether what you speak can impact your thought process. Your language could shape your reality, so have a think about whether you need to change your narrative.

Do you open your mouth, and the words spill out without much thought about the impact of what you're saying to your audience, or do you choose your words wisely and rehearse ahead of time?

You could try recording your conversations, to get a better view of the language you use. The other aspect to this, is the language used by others and how their cohesive language can result in you having a change in mood.

Look at our questioning techniques section in the coaching element of the support chapter. It's my belief that language used by yourself, and others can impact on your wellbeing affecting your mood negatively or positively.

Major Life Changes

Experience shows us that many life changing moments such as ill health, divorce, birth of a child, loss of loved ones, redundancy or moving home can result in us having a dip in our own wellbeing and can lead to heightened levels of stress, anxiety, and depression.

Most people have experienced a roller coaster ride through life and human behaviour shows that we naturally prefer having a routine, so when this change happens, that is out of our control, it can take us out of our comfort zones and have an impact on our mental health.

The best way to understand this is by looking at the **'Kubler-Ross Grief Cycle model'**, (Kubler-Ross, E. and Kessler, D., 2005). This is commonly known as the grief cycle, with five different stages:

This process is not necessarily linear, and it could be that you experience the various stages in different orders or that you experience a number of the stages at the same time?

The denial stage is a survival mechanism whereby you are living in your preferred reality rather than the actual reality.

The Kubler-Ross Grief Cycle

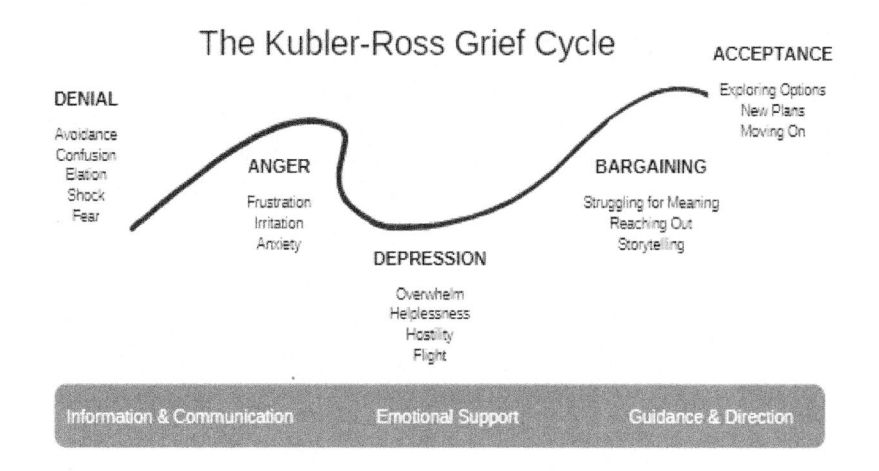

DENIAL
Avoidance
Confusion
Elation
Shock
Fear

ANGER
Frustration
Irritation
Anxiety

DEPRESSION
Overwhelm
Helplessness
Hostility
Flight

BARGAINING
Struggling for Meaning
Reaching Out
Storytelling

ACCEPTANCE
Exploring Options
New Plans
Moving On

Information & Communication | Emotional Support | Guidance & Direction

The anger stage is a natural and a necessary stage of grief, you need to go through this stage for it to leave you, it can cause you to question your values and beliefs in many things like your faith or humanity. It is a natural part of the healing process.

The bargaining stage is about us trying to skip through the grief and regain normality again by making promises to ourselves about making dramatic changes that are hard to achieve. It is important to have awareness of when you are going through the bargaining stage, so you're realistic about what you can achieve.

The depression stage is about having an awareness of your emotions following a grief event. It's often because of feeling emotionally overwhelmed.

Acceptance is when you have recognised why things have happened and you're able to move forward. This may require you to have a readjustment of your life and circumstances, however you are more likely to have more better days than bad and adjust to your new reality.

The thing is, it is perfectly normal and what makes us human, we go from being in denial, to anger, to detaching ourselves and withdrawing, to telling our story, to acceptance and then moving forward to a meaningful life again. This happens to everybody, and it helps to take comfort in that.

There are some people that prefer novelty and spontaneity and there are things we can learn from these people that can help us thrive in the most major of life changes. Here are a few tips to help you reframe your mind and look at things in a slightly different way:

- ♥ Positive changes can also bring along dips in our wellbeing, due to fear of the unknown and it is important to embrace this and acknowledge that this is perfectly normal too.

- ♥ Use strategies to help you manage your stresses, everyone is different so it's a case of finding the right outlet for you to improve your wellbeing, see early chapters in this book. Create new routines that bring your joy and happiness.

- ♥ When life changing events happen it brings uncertainty, this bias is a natural part of life and once you can recognise this, you can then move forward rationally and start to see things more positively.

- ♥ Use the IF-THEN rule, you can use this to help you find alternative ways of moving forward. So, IF this happens then I could THEN do this. You will be amazed at how many positive alternatives you can come up with.

- ♥ Continue to work on your resilience, if you have had life changing events, think back on how you dealt with that and find your coping mechanisms and implement them now.

- ♥ Look at the life changing event as an opportunity to start a new page in your life. It could give you the chance to try something that you have always wanted to do, and it is important to practise self-care and reward or treat yourself and celebrate the wins however big they are.

- ♥ Devise a new plan, at first things may be a little disorganised, this is because you're finding your way and trying new things, once you have a firmer routine in place then you can move towards making stronger plans.

- ♥ Reach out to others, this could be for 1-2-1 support, or it could be joining a new class or starting a new hobby or job, reach out to your network and see what is out there to help you move forward.

Innovation

For some people the word innovation means moving out of their comfort zone and is a catalyst for change and you would be exactly right.

The definition of innovation concerns the implementation of fresh ideas, and I hope the earlier chapters in this book will have helped you to reframe your mind into, thinking about innovation in a more positive light, as a way of helping you grow as a person, in helping you to be successful in your stretch zone and hopefully help you to achieve your full potential whatever that looks like for you.

During the pandemic, we have all been through incredible amounts of change and I can imagine you would have had an opportunity to learn several new skills?

Much was out of our control due to government restrictions, but it's a terrific idea to reflect on how well you have done and think about how you can use that learning to be more like that person now we are gradually returning to some kind of normal existence.

Change is one certainty in life and in the future things will continue to change, just think how much more you will be valued if you're able to be a more rounded person, open to these changes both in terms of your career and in your home life?

The job market is changing and because of this many people are looking to retrain and try something new, those more sustainable businesses, will already be making plans to diversify the type of roles that they recruit for.

Innovation in the workplace

Innovation is often described as one of three things: radical/disruptive innovation, incremental innovation, or a blend of both depending on the organisation and scope, time, and resource of the project.

Disruptive Innovation can be described as when a particular industry gets shaken up.

Incremental innovation is a series of small improvements or upgrades made to a company's existing products, services, processes, or methods.

Whatever career you choose, Innovation will be embedded as part of everyday strategy. So how can you lead these changes and influence others?

Here are some ideas for you to consider:

- ♥ Start your own enterprise based on your passions
- ♥ Having high levels of energy, any innovation takes time to come to fruition, so keep energy high and build a sense of enthusiasm for fresh ideas within your team.
- ♥ Encourage creativity. Doing things that you have always done will always lead to the same results, so give yourself and others thinking time and actively capture new ideas. Creativity workshops could be a great way to do this as could fracturing in time within your week, to work on new projects and experiment with these new ideas.
- ♥ Be part of a positive culture, With the huge transformation you have undergone since reading this book, you could be that positive influence in

creating the right culture that nurtures creativity and innovation. Recognise that failures are never failures and use it as a learning opportunity. You could also use this opportunity to fine tune new ways of working that could help you stand out among your peers and colleagues.

- ♥ Embrace your differences. If you are looking for a new job role because of the pandemic, how about moving into a completely new field or industry. The benefits you can take to your new role, could help transform their traditional policies and procedures. This could be a fantastic way of helping them see things differently and help them to see things with a fresh pair of eyes. What a way of making a positive impact.

All businesses, whether they are products or services, go on a journey of life cycle, quite often they start with innovation and over time they can become mature, and it is the businesses that innovate that stand the test of time and move forward with fresh ideas and reinvent themselves.

I would ask you to think about yourself in this scenario and compare yourself to the life cycle. Have you reached maturity and is it time to stretch yourself and move into a new role or career? You have mastered your skill so is it time for you to now step up and move into a different role?

Burnout to Bold

My Ditty: The face of a clown

'My Goodness why was I being pulled into this again?', I groaned internally. It was that time of year, when a working group of a cross section of staff were asked to form a team and arrange this year's Annual Conference.

'Marie, we have arranged the team and need you to drive everyone over to the Safari Park', were the words that rang in my head. Our CEO was standing in front of me, how could I possibly say NO?

'Yes, sure', were the words coming out of my mouth, yet inside, I was in turmoil. "No way, do you not know that I am up to my eyes in work at the moment with deadlines to meet" was my inner voice.

Why, could I not just say at that time, that I needed my workload reviewing, if I was to get involved in this Conference this year? In simple terms, the reality was that I respected my CEO, and it was well known that he didn't take kindly to people saying they were Busy.

We all got on board the minibus and it was a fantastic atmosphere. The team had a wealth of ideas of how this year's conference was going to be the best one yet. We were shown around the venue, which was just like a big top circus tent, and then we were ushered into the cafe to discuss our ideas along with the CEO.

He posed the question, 'So what do you think now you have seen the venue, what could we do to make this the best conference to date?', I told myself before we went that I was just going to be a spectator and that I was only the driver. I needed to remain quiet.

It was like tumbleweed, all the enthusiasm that had created such a brilliant atmosphere in the minibus had vanished into thin air. Everyone just looked at each other without a word being uttered. The CEO remained quiet and sipped on his coffee whilst his question just hung in the air.

My eyes scanned around the team and all I saw were

blank faces, "Please someone say something", was my inner voice. We sat there for what seemed like an eternity and the silence was becoming deafening. I looked over at the CEO and I sensed that he was becoming frustrated.

'Please anyone, just say something, anything'. Again, my inner voice was urging someone to say something". Again, silence was dominating the space.

'How about we use the fantastic venue and do something along the theme of a Circus?', I had to break the silence, and although I promised myself, I was not going to contribute. I thought by starting the conversation, it would help people to chip in and alleviate the frustration of our CEO, that I could sense was getting crosser by the moment.

'Great idea, and we could dress up as clowns?', Phew the conversation had started. Then what followed was the team creativity with lots of Innovate ideas that was going to make this the best Conference yet.

When I reflect on my involvement, I recognise that I showed Leadership, by empowering the team to feel that they had great ideas and all contributions were valid.

Was my fixed mindset helpful when my CEO approached me?

Through great teamwork and innovation, we delivered a brilliant 'Circus' themed conference. Did we dress as clowns? Yes, absolutely, in fact we made our own costumes, and all looked the part.

The important point here is that by having a working group from a cross section of the organisation, we were able to address the cultural issues raised through the staff surveys at the conference and influence positive changes, which was a win-win situation to find ourselves in.

Burnout to Bold

Burnout to Bold

CHAPTER 8 : LEADERSHIP

Are Leaders born or are they Made? Can anyone be a leader? Are you a leader? These are just a few of the questions that I explored when I started my own business back in 2015 after my recovery. Since then, I have come to understand leadership in various ways.

Leadership: Well as I see it, anyone can be a Leader, you do not need to have a fancy title to be a leader. You can find Leadership in a cross section of an organisation and in society. Some people will naturally have leadership skills based on their upbringing and others will go and learn the skills to become a leader.

There can also be the element of being in the right place at the right time. As history has shown us, not all leaders get it right, all the time, and it is important to appreciate that leaders are human too. The point here is that if you want to become a leader then you absolutely could, it requires dedication, commitment to learning, practise and experience.

There are certain attributes that you will find in leadership:

- **Integrity:** Having a strong moral compass and being honest can set you apart from others, people will have confidence in you to do the right thing for them and for the business.

- **Charisma:** Charismatic leaders are often magnetic and have a certain charm about themselves and can inspire others to be the best versions of themselves.

- **Vision**: If you're the type of person that can impart wisdom and have imagination of how things could look, then you could be a visionary.

- **Positivity**: If you can see positives in any situation, then people are likely to gravitate towards you and if you're optimistic then it helps to motivate others.

- ♥ **Great Communicator**: Communication is key to a successful leadership and is probably the most important attribute. This includes listening, speaking, observing, and having empathy for others.

These are just a few of the attributes that can define a leader, although there are many more like confidence, dynamic, inspiring, effective team builder, foresight and identify opportunities.

The best book I have read on Leadership has to be, **'The 7 Habits of Highly Effective People'**, by Stephen Covey. In this book Covey helps leaders or inspiring leaders to move from dependency to independence and or interdependence by practicing 7 habits.

Leadership Styles

Every leader has an inherent style that they favour, although there are times when it can improve a situation or scenario to alter your style and it might be that you adapt your leadership style based on the audience. The best way to lead is to understand yourself better and this will help you to become a better and more inspiring leader.

The Harvard Business Review has carried out extensive research into what these styles are:

> **https://hbr.org/2005/04/seven-transformations-of-leadership**

1. **Opportunist:** can bring about transformation in the current way of working and they can create an appealing environment that enables other work colleagues to pursue certain risks.

2. **Diplomat:** makes sense of the world around them in a more harmonised way; they tend to focus on gaining control of one's own behaviour. Diplomats provide social glue to their colleagues and ensure that attention is paid to the needs of others.

3. **Expert:** try to exercise control by perfecting their knowledge, both in their professional and personal lives. They are more likely to present hard data and logic in their efforts to gain consensus and buy-in from others.

4. **Achiever**: these leaders influence and create a positive work environment and focus their efforts on deliverables, they are open to feedback and are aware of sensitivity in relationships.

5. **Individualist:** they put personalities and ways of relating into perspective and communicate well with people who have other leadership styles to them. They tend to follow their own path.

6. **Strategist:** their focus is also adept at creating shared visions across all leadership styles. They encourage both personal and organisational transformations, they're better at handling people's instinctive resistance to change.

7. **Alchemist**: they have an ability to renew or even reinvent themselves and they have an extraordinary capacity to deal simultaneously with many situations at multiple levels and with different people regardless of their seniority. They can deal with immediate priorities yet never lose sight of long-term goals.

You can take the Leadership Development profile test on numerous websites, or you could work with a business coach or executive coach to explore this further.

> **I would recommend Marie Haycocks from Certanovo if you want to work with a coach to develop your Leadership skills.**
> https://certanovo.com/about.html

Leadership Voices

'**Every leader has their own voice**', (Detert, J. and Burris, E., 2007.). When I say this, I don't mean how they vocalise a message, I am referring to the values and communication skills to empower and inspire others.

Leaders must be deliberate about articulating their values and living by them. This requires you to maintain your confidence and ensure that imposter syndrome does not creep in.

The other consideration is likeability. As a leader you need to free yourself from the need to be liked, otherwise you can end up being more concerned with being a people pleaser over taking honest feedback and building your leadership skills.

The reality is, there will be times when you lead, that will require you to make strategic decisions that are not fully understood by most of the team, and you will be questioned about your decision making.

You will need to be able to face this without being coerced into changing your decisions, although it is also important to remain flexible. Sometimes leaders have to take a stance to achieve a greater good for the many, not just the few.

We mentioned earlier in this chapter about charismatic leadership, and this is where likeability is a factor. You can be liked as a leader and it is important to be able to show kindness, forgiveness, humility and remain humble. It is a balancing act, that not all leaders get right, however it is useful to be aware of these characteristics to be a better leader.

Characteristics

As a leader it is important to be ethical, and your character, your ability to delegate and how you empower others should be key ingredients of your leadership approach.

We have picked up on numerous characteristics, attributes, and styles of leadership earlier in this chapter although there are other characteristics that could help you become an inspirational leader.

> **Visit our website for our FREE downloadable 'Leadership Strengths Handout':**
>
> **Our website is**
> **www.advanceyourwellbeing.co.uk**

Empowering

Having courage is something that requires you to be bold in your decision making and it also requires you to have courage and trust in others. Those workforces that are empowered are more likely to have higher job satisfaction. So why is empowerment such an important characteristic for leaders?

Instilling confidence in your peers and colleagues is one of the best gifts you can give, it helps to build trust, it creates ownership and accountability and aids personal responsibility. The other thing to consider here is that leaders are at risk of micro-managing, and this can cause burn out, so there are personal benefits to leadership to create an empowering environment.

Authenticity

The reality is that people buy people and workforces want leaders that are real and authentic. Authenticity emphasises building the leader's legitimacy through honest relationships. While workforces recognise the importance of having access to performance data based on sales and profitability, it is not the key driver for individuals in today's society.

Authentic leadership is a refreshing alternative to historic leadership. People are looking for leaders that have a social consciousness and when you're authentic and looking at the impact of your organisation on the community at large, you are more likely to be able to attract the best talent out there.

Inspiration

There are many people in history that you can class as inspirational, and everyone has different views on what they believe is inspirational.

Can you be your own inspiration? By studying people, you admire and looking at their attributes, characteristics, and achievements, ask yourself what it is that you admire and what could you learn and replicate yourself?

Self-Inspiration

You are the only one who knows what you are truly capable of and how willing you are to push yourself. You are the only person who can change your mindset and evoke change in the areas of your life you want to improve.

Is it healthy to compare yourself to others to gain the motivation to achieve your full potential? It could be far healthier and better for your wellbeing, to follow your own path and focus inwards?

Life has many ups and downs, and we all need inspiration from time to time, and while people have been used as inspirational figures through the generations, you can gain inspiration in other forms, Music, Quotes, Art, Faith, Nature, Books and many more. You just need to find what it is that inspires you to achieve your goals.

My Ditty: Let's do this...

After months of applying for numerous jobs online, with little success. I recognised that I needed to do something positive with my life. How could it be that I had achieved promotion after promotion in my Housing role, and successfully led a number of teams and been recognised with a prestigious accreditation in Housing, yet I couldn't get a job as a receptionist or a cafe?

Was it my honesty about having been out of work for a year with poor mental health that was making me unemployable?

All these questions had to stop, I needed to put my hand into something that was going to make me feel like I had a purpose and help me to stretch into my growth zone.

I recognised that I could use what had been a negative part of my life to help others and hopefully make a positive difference to them. I then took the important step to start my own business and lead by example.

I sat there with my laptop in front of me. 'Right, Let's do this...', was my positive mindset and my inner voice was generating a myriad of questions. What would my offering be, what would I call my business, who could I help and add value too?

Once I had made the commitment to start my own business, I found the motivation and determination to go for it, 100%. My confidence & self-esteem was still building, after months and months of personal development following my lowest ebb when I considered taking my own life. I knew that to be a leader again, I needed to explore further my strengths and areas to improve.

I joined a ladies-only networking group, which was a group of wonderful businesswomen that inspired me to feel that I could achieve a successful business. This is where I met a lady called Tracey Powiesnik from Core Process. She explained how she helps people to create leadership styles that are inclusive, confident, and transparent.

I automatically thought, her help was just what I needed in my Leadership journey. It was hugely insightful. I completed an online assessment and arranged to meet in person to explore the results.

After meeting with Tracey, it gave me a boost to my self-esteem, I knew that I had areas to improve and thought with practise and more learning. I could absolutely do this.

Burnout to Bold

Burnout to Bold

CHAPTER 9 : SUPPORT COACHING

Today there seems to be a rise in popularity in having a coach to help and support you to achieve your goals and dreams. There are different coaching roles so it's useful to understand what types there are and how they can help.

Wellbeing Coaches: They take a holistic approach to helping their clients live a positive and fulfilled life. Rather than concentrate on just one area, they work with their clients to identify specific issues in all areas of their life.

Fitness Coaches: They are professional in the field of fitness and exercise and combine the coaching process with personal training. They help to develop and maintain personal fit lifestyles.

Career Coaches: focus on the current situation and create action goals to help clients move forward in their career. They help you make informed decisions about your career development and trajectory.

Leadership Coaches: This is a coach that helps leaders or potential leaders design a bespoke development plan through a process of inviting introspection and self-reflection that helps them to tap into their full potential.

Strategic Coaches: Strategy is complex and having a coach who specialises in facilitating the process of defining customer focus, analysing market needs, and developing strategic plans can help structure and accelerate business processes. As well as helping with Business Plans, they can help stakeholders communicate and implement that plan.

Team Coaches: Team coaches focus on helping define a team's purpose, set goals, clarify roles and responsibilities, and work through interpersonal dynamics

Executive Coaches: They provide a safe, structured, and trustworthy environment in which to offer support for individuals be it a CEO, Executive Directors, Middle-Management, Governance and Board Members, with a particular focus on improving performance and behaviour in the workplace.

Business Coaches: for support in all areas of building your business from creating a solid admin foundation through to developing the skills you need for success.

I recommend you read, **'Love Coaching, Hate Business'**, by Ali Bagley & Susan Lane, two amazing business coaches. In this book they give you everything you need to get the business side of your coaching practice up and running.

Now you have a better understanding of the type of coach you need, it is worth understanding that every coach has a different style, and you will have to find the right one for you.

Here are some of the key elements that you should look for in a coach:

People oriented: People naturally feel comfortable in their company

Font of knowledge: With vast experience and knowledge.

Effective communicator: They listen well and explain things in a clear and understandable way.

Supporter: They enjoy supporting people even if that means sometimes being firm and asking hard questions.

Dedicated: An individual who is dedicated to helping you succeed.

Certified / Accredited: They are well trained and can prove their ability to work well with you.

What is coaching?

It is important to note that a coach is not a mentor, councillor, therapist, or a consultant. A coach's main job is to help the individual realise for themselves what they want to achieve by looking at future possibilities, by listening and using powerful questioning techniques.

Their main purpose is to empower the individual to go on a journey of self-discovery, improve their own effectiveness and help to gain clarity over time.

Questioning techniques

The most effective coaches are masters of questioning techniques. It is useful to understand a bit more about the different types of questions that can be used, with a few examples. You can look out for them.

Type of Question	Description	Example
Open	Generally encourages wider discussion and elaboration.	What do you think about XYZ? Why did you choose that item?
Closed	Requires a one-word answer, such as 'yes' or 'no'.	Do you like X? Have you taken the X?
Fact Based	Searches for information.	What is your name? Would you like X, Y or Z?
Probing	A series of questions that dig deeper and provide a fuller picture.	When do you need the finished project? Is it ok if I send this to you?
Statement	Require a yes or no answer. Statement questions are about making a statement with a question mark.	That is your X? She did that before?
Leading	Lead the respondent towards a certain desired route.	Did you enjoy? Do you have any issues with this?

Funnel	Begin broadly before narrowing to a specific point	What do you do? Followed by another question like, Why did you choose to be an X?'
Recall	Require the recipient to remember a fact.	Where did you put the X? What is ten x ten?
Process	Require the coach to add their own opinion to their answer. These types of questions could be used to test depth of knowledge about a particular topic.	Why are you the right person to lead this project? What are the benefits of changing the process of X?

I hope that this helps you have an insight into what types of questions that your coach could use, to enable you to build a robust relationship with your coach and gain a better understanding of how these questions could be used to help you along the process. Special mention to Alan C Clark the management whisper for coaching me along my business journey.

After reading this chapter, it might inspire you to learn more about coaching and I could recommend The Coaching Academy, because it could be helpful for you in your future job role whatever your position in an organisation.

Further information about this can be found on The Coaching Academy website:

https://www.the-coaching-academy.com/

Coaching Models

Different coaches will use different coaching models to

support your growth and it could be worth asking what model your coach uses to find the best fit for you. All models are similar in nature with the desired outcome of supporting you to achieve your full potential.

Here is an example of the **GROW model** (J, Whitmore):

G: - Goal

R: - Currently Reality

O: - Options

W: - Will or Way forward

The model was originally developed in the 1980s by business coaches Graham Alexander, Alan Fine, and Sir John Whitmore. A good way of thinking about the GROW Model is to think about how you would plan a journey.

First, you decide where you are going (the goal) and establish where you currently are (your current reality). You then explore various routes (the options) to your destination.

In the final step, establishing the will, you ensure that you're committed to making the journey, and are prepared for the obstacles that you could meet on the way.

What is Mentoring?

A mentor is a person with more knowledge or experience in a particular field then the mentee. This is regardless of age or gender. A mentor often takes a holistic approach to providing support in numerous areas to the mentee.

You do not need to have a qualification to become a mentor but a passion to help others is vital. You can have a mentor in your personal life or in a business setting.

A great book to read is, **'The Mentoring Manual: Step by step guide to being a better mentor'**, by Julia Starr or the **'Mentoring Mindset: Skills and tools'**, by Anne Rolfe

This relationship is about supporting the mentee in increasing in confidence and empowerment, by gaining additional knowledge and taking ownership of their own development. So, what is a mentor?

- ♥ Someone who can provide advice on personal development or knowledge-based skills.
- ♥ An active listener, someone with excellent communication skills.
- ♥ Someone with experience. It is useful to understand different people's insights in how they overcame challenges.
- ♥ Someone who encourages you to do self-reflection. How else can you become more self-aware?
- ♥ A non-judgemental sounding-board. It's useful to bounce ideas around. Sharing ideas can help you improve on what your original thought process was. Finding better solutions or innovation
- ♥ An introducer to networks and contacts. Diversity can help enrich your ideas and perspectives. Along with the possibility of new opportunities.
- ♥ Someone who empowers others. By mentoring someone you are there to encourage responsibility and accountability. You as the mentor are facilitating the process.
- ♥ Gives career advice. This can be through looking at your weaknesses or areas for development and most importantly your strengths.

Mentoring or Coaching?

It is important to note that a coach and a mentor fulfil different functions. It is worth putting some thought into what role you need to support you. It could even be that both roles are what is needed.

My Ditty: Jumping for joy

I pulled on my red running pants and ran out towards the Gym. Today's PE lesson was Trampolining. I always enjoyed taking part in all sports in school, from Netball, cross-country running to rounders. Today, Miss Evans was going to take us for Trampolining.

As a little girl, when we went to the seaside, my brother and I would always go and jump for 3 minutes on the fair ground trampolines. I can always remember the one at Ragley Hall too which was part of the outdoor adventure park. We would nag our nan and grandad to let us have a play.

I liked the idea of learning how to jump and do the tricks and I always looked forward to Miss Evans PE and Games lessons. Her approach to teaching new skills was one that I valued as a young girl. She always made it seem possible that we could excel at anything we put our minds to.

"Marie it is your turn", after waiting patiently for my turn, I clambered up onto the huge Olympic size trampoline. There was a red cross in the middle of the canvas, and I was guided to start jumping on the spot. Woohoo, I jumped and jumped and was thrust up into the air.

I thought I would touch the Gym ceiling, I was reaching such great heights, it was completely different from the childhood experience of trampolining on the fairground ones.

After weeks of learning to trampoline in PE, Miss Evens decided to start an after-school club. I was first in the queue to put my name on the list. Then on our first day, she explained that we would be taking part in school championships and that we needed to learn a routine.

Thinking back, I was completely up for the opportunity. Her coaching style, and nurturing nature always got results. She was one of those ladies that inspired us as young girls. Such a positive influence.

We went on as a team to win various medals at the Championships. I got a bronze medal and while it was not silver or gold. I felt proud of our whole team's achievement. It was always about celebrating individual and team progress and working towards improvements, rather than the win.

Miss Evans was fantastic at her job, as a teacher and coach and she knew exactly how to get the best out of us. This is what the right coach can do for you, so whatever it is you want to achieve then it is well worth reaching out to a coach, it can mean the difference between having an idea or being successful.

Burnout to BOLD

Burnout to BOLD

AND FINALLY

I hope you found the pick and mix of topics that helped me on my journey from facing the possibility of ending my life to first rate wellbeing, as well as being a bold entrepreneur, of use?

And did you enjoy my real-life ditties? Stories from my past that have dramatically shaped my life that I hope will have resonated with your own experiences.

Thank you for reading my book. Now it's your turn to take the bull by the horns and achieve your full potential. You are in charge of your life; you just need to believe in your dreams.

Now go for it and be **BOLD.**

Appendices

Supplementary Resources

available on my website:
www.advanceyourwellbeing.co.uk

5 Ways to Wellbeing Booklet

This booklet could help you to achieve your Wellbeing goals, using each of the steps of this model.

What Wellbeing Means To Me Handout

This handout helps you to think about and identify what Wellbeing means to you.

Health Check Handout

Using this handout will help you to identify bad habits and change them to healthier and positive changes.

Reflection Handout

Use reflection to get in touch with your emotions and give yourself the space you need to capture them.

My Gratitude Notes

Identify things in your life that you're grateful for and take a note to help to practise mindfulness and emotional intelligence.

Pledge Card

By keeping a record of your promises, you're more likely to achieve them.

Childhood: My personal experiences Handout

Often in life we are moving from one experience to another. This handout gives you an opportunity to see what has shaped you in your life.

Values and Beliefs to Positive Behaviour Handout

Self-awareness of our own values and beliefs is something that can help you to make positive change behaviours. This handout will help you with this.

Mindset test

This is an opportunity to assess what type of mindset you have and change it if you need to.

Leadership Strengths Handout

We all have the capability to be a leader, this handout helps to identify your strengths and areas to build on.

Bibliography: Books mentioned or recommended

An Examination Of Our Own Extraordinariness by Howard, E, Gardener

Eat that Frog by Brian Tracy

Emotional Intelligence: Why it can matter more than IQ by Daniel Goleman

Emotional Intelligence 2.0 by Jean Greaves and Travis Bradberry

Extraordinary Minds: Portraits Of 4 Exceptional Individuals by Howard, E, Gardener

How to be an Adult in Relationships by David Ricoh

Love Coaching, Hate Business by Ali Bagley & Susan Lane

Men are from Mars and Women are from Venus by John Gray

The Mentoring Manual: Step by step guide to being a better mentor by Julia Starr

Mentoring Mindset: Skills and tools by Anne Rolfe

Mindfulness and Mental Health by Chris Mace

Mindfulness by Prof Mark Williams & Dr Danny Penman

Mindset; The new psychology of success by Prof Carol Dweck

No Such Thing as Normal by Bryony Gordon

Reinventing Organisations by Frederic Laloux

Resilient by Rick Hanson

Resilient Me by Sam Owen

Resilience for Today: Gaining strength in adversity by Edith Henderson Grotberg

The child's right to play: A global approach by Rhonda L Clements and Leah Fiorentino.

The Chimp Paradox by Steven Peters

The Little Teal Book of Trust by Jeffrey Gitomer

The Resilience Club by Angela Armstrong

The Success Cycle: 3 Keys for Achieving Your Goals in Business and Life by Marques Ogden.

The 7 Habits of Highly Effective People by Stephen Covey.

Other Sources
Marie Jenkins Advance your Wellbeing
https://www.youtube.com/channel/UCZr9PEY30avgHClqnw3d0Ig
Jenkins Journey Blogs
https://jenkinsjourneys.tumblr.com/
Ernie Said
http://www.erniesaid.info/

https://www.youtube.com/watch?v=uI3L9rCRWkY
Joe Wicks: The body coach
https://www.youtube.com/user/thebodycoach1
The Mental Health Foundation
https://www.mentalhealth.org.uk/

https://www.mentalhealth.org.uk/blog/importance-sleep

https://www.mentalhealth.org.uk/publications/how-to-using-exercise
TED ED- Dunning-Kruger Effect
https://www.ted.com/talks/david_dunning_why_incompetent_people_think_they_re_amazing/transcript?language=en
Emotional Intelligence - Daniel Goleman
https://www.danielgoleman.info
Trust Equation - Hannah Price
https://blog.jostle.me/blog/ways-to-build-trust-at-work
Coaching Questioning Techniques
https://www.mindtools.com/pages/article/newTMC_88.htm
Gig Economy
https://www.youtube.com/watch?v=oQfTJy0sRVs

MIND Charity

https://www.mind.org.uk/

www.mind.org.uk/information-support/tips-for-everyday-living/nature-and-mental-health/about-ecotherapy-programmes/

TEDx Talk from Elizabeth McClure

https://www.youtube.com/watch?v=g00o6LCmaMI

Lisa Billingham Author of Katie: The new chapter

https://m.facebook.com/100664191733679/photos/a.102394328227332/200508021749295/?type=3&_rdr

Adrianne Carter The Face Whisperer

https://adriannecarter.com/

Marie Haycocks from Certanovo

https://certanovo.com/about.html

Alan C Clark The Management Whisperer

https://www.keybiz.com/

The Coaching Academy

https://www.the-coaching-academy.com/

References

2021. Looking after your Mental Health using exercise. 1st ed. [e-book] The Mental Health Foundation. Available at: https://www.mentalhealth.org.uk/sites/default/files/How%20to...exercise.pdf [Accessed 10 June 2021].

Association of psychological science. 2011. Research States That Prejudice Comes From a Basic Human Need and Way of Thinking. [online] Available at: https://www.psychologicalscience.org/news/releases/research-states-that-prejudice-comes-from-a-basic-human-need-and-way-of-thinking.html [Accessed 23 June 2021].

Atlas Biomed blog | Take control of your health with no-nonsense news on lifestyle, gut microbes and genetics. 2021. Serotonin And The Other Happy Hormones In Your Body. [online] Available at: https://atlasbiomed.com/blog/serotonin-and-other-happy-molecules-made-by-gut-bacteria/ [Accessed 24 June 2021].

Bhf.org.uk. 2021. Feeling stressed? Research shows how stress can lead to heart attacks and stroke. [online] Available at: https://www.bhf.org.uk/informationsupport/heart-matters-magazine/news/behind-the-headlines/stress-and-heart-disease [Accessed 21 June 2021].

Detert, J. and Burris, E., 2007. Leadership Behaviour and Employee Voice: Is the door really open? Academy of Management Journal, [online] 50(4). Available at: https://journals.aom.org/doi/abs/10.5465/AMJ.2007.26279183 [Accessed 16 June 2021].

Gills, B. (2006) Accepting Difference, Finding Tolerance, Practising Dialogue, Globalizations, 3:4, 423-426, DOI: 10.1080/14747730601121909

Gologor, E. (1977). On accepting diversity. American Psychologist, 32(11), 986–987. https://doi.org/10.1037/0003-066X.32.11.986

GOV.UK. 2008. Five ways to mental wellbeing. [online] Available at: https://www.gov.uk/government/publications/five-ways-to-mental-wellbeing [Accessed 14 June 2021].

Healthline. 2021. How Much Water Should You Drink Per Day? [online] Available at: https://www.healthline.com/nutrition/how-much-water-should-you-drink-per-day [Accessed 24 June 2021].

Higgins, D. (2011) Why reflect? Recognising the link between learning and reflection, Reflective Practice, 12:5, 583-584, DOI: 10.1080/14623943.2011.606693

Kubler-Ross, E. and Kessler, D., 2005. On grief and Grieving:Finding the meaning of grief through the five stages of loss. 1st ed. New York: Simon and Schuster.

Marshall, L., 2020. Emerging evidence on COVID-19's impact on mental health and health inequalities | The Health Foundation. [online] The Health Foundation. Available at: https://www.health.org.uk/news-and-comment/blogs/emerging-evidence-on-covid-19s-impact-on-mental-health-and-health?gclid=EAIaIQobChMI68jEqPq66wIVnIBQBh3YuADIEAAYASAAEgIXifD_BwE [Accessed 10 June 2021].

Maslow, A., 2021. Maslow's Hierarchy of Needs – Research History. [online] Researchhistory.org. Available at: http://www.researchhistory.org/2012/06/16/maslows-hierarchy-of-needs/?print=1 [Accessed 14 June 2021].

Mathias, G., 2021. 5 Pillars of resilience | Gill Mathias. [online] Gillmathias.com. Available at: https://gillmathias.com/category/5-pillars-of-resilience/#:~:text=5%20Pillars%20of%20resilience%20

%7C%20Gill%20Mathias [Accessed 14 June 2021].

Mental Health Foundation. 2021. How to look after your mental health using exercise. [online] Available at: https://www.mentalhealth.org.uk/publications/how-to-using-exercise#:~:text=It%20is%20recommended%20that%20the,or%20skipping%20with%20a%20rope. [Accessed 21 June 2021].

Mind.org.uk. 2018. About ecotherapy programmes. [online] Available at: https://www.mind.org.uk/information-support/tips-for-everyday-living/nature-and-mental-health/about-ecotherapy-programmes/#:~:text=Ecotherapy%20is%20a%20formal%20type,are%20there%20to%20support%20you [Accessed 14 June 2021].

Mitchel, A., 2016. Burnout and the Brain. [online] Association for Psychological Science - APS. Available at: https://www.psychologicalscience.org/observer/burnout-and-the-brain [Accessed 24 June 2021].

Noble T., McGrath H. (2012) Wellbeing and Resilience in Young People and the Role of Positive Relationships. In: Roffey S. (eds) Positive Relationships. Springer, Dordrecht. https://doi.org/10.1007/978-94-007-2147-0_2

Oxford Mindfulness Centre. 2021. About Us - Oxford Mindfulness Centre. [online] Available at: https://www.oxfordmindfulness.org/ [Accessed 23 June 2021].

Rinard, M., 2021. Living in the comfort zone | ACM SIGPLAN Notices. [online] Dl.acm.org. Available at: https://dl.acm.org/doi/abs/10.1145/1297105.1297072 [Accessed 14 June 2021].

Rooke, D. and Torbert, W., 2005. Seven Transformations

of Leadership. Harvard Business Review, [online] Available at: https://hbr.org/2005/04/seven-transformations-of-leadership [Accessed 16 June 2021].

Saltzman, L., Hansel, T. and Bordnick, P., 2020. Loneliness, isolation, and Social Support Factors in post COVID 19 Mental Health. 1st ed. New Orleans: Tulane University.

Sterrett, E., 2014. Assessing Emotional Intelligence. Amherst: HRD Press, https://downloads.hrdpressonline.com/files/2520140310180218.pdf

Sciaraffa, M.A., Zeanah, P.D. & Zeanah, C.H. Understanding and Promoting Resilience in the Context of Adverse Childhood Experiences. Early Childhood Educ J 46, 343–353 (2018). https://doi.org/10.1007/s10643-017-0869-3

Sidhu, and Deletraz, 2015. Effect of Comfort Zone on Entrepreneurship Potential, Innovation Culture, and Career Satisfaction. 1st ed. [e-book] Seattle. Available at: http://file:///ASEE_CZ_Paper_Final_2.9.1.pdf [Accessed 14 June 2021].

Tseng, J., Poppenk, J. 2020. Brain meta-state transitions demarcate thoughts across task contexts exposing the mental noise of trait neuroticism. Nat Commun 11, 3480 (2020). https://doi.org/10.1038/s41467-020-17255-9

Wardekker, W. (1998) Scientific Concepts and Reflection, Mind, Culture, and Activity, 5:2, 143-153, DOI: 10.1207/s15327884mca0502_8

White, A., 2008. From Comfort Zone to Performance Management. 1st ed. Baisy-Thy: White and Maclean Publishing.Whitney Gibson, J., Greenwood, R. A., & Murphy, Jr., E. F. (2009). Generational Differences In The Workplace: Personal Values, Behaviours, And Popular Beliefs. Journal of Diversity Management (JDM), 4(3), 1-

8. https://doi.org/10.19030/jdm.v4i3.4959

Woods-Jaegar, B., Cho, B. and Sexton, C., 2018. Promoting Resilience: Breaking the Intergenerational Cycle of Adverse Childhood Experiences - Briana A. Woods-Jaeger, Bridget Cho, Chris C. Sexton, Lauren Slagel, Kathy Goggin, 2018. [online] SAGE Journals. Available at: https://journals.sagepub.com/doi/abs/10.1177/1090198117752785 [Accessed 14 June 2021].

BURNOUT TO BOLD

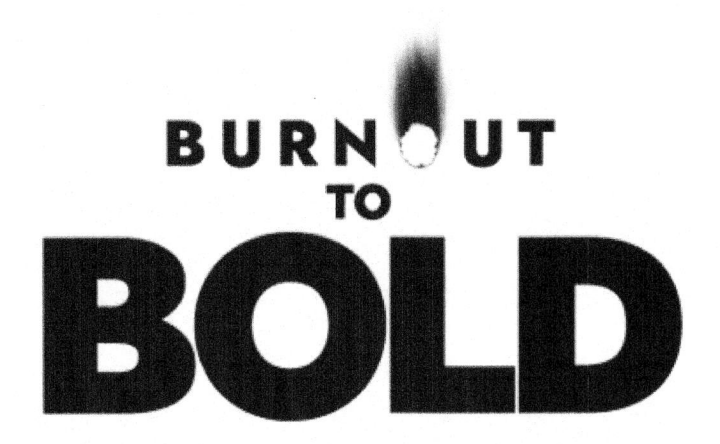

From a flickering light to a bold flame

Marie Jenkins

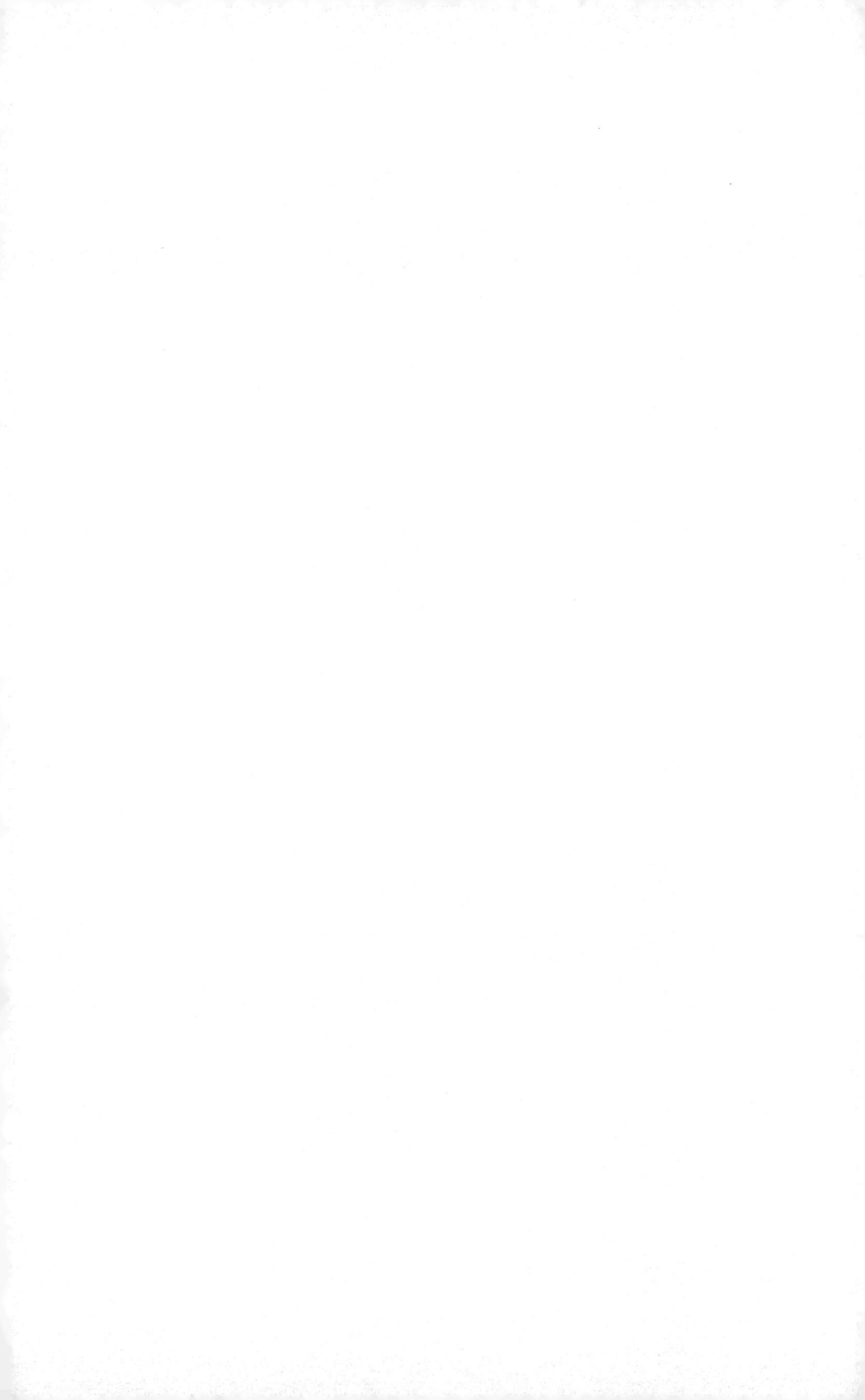

Printed in Great Britain
by Amazon